THIS is Dyslexia

THIS is Dyslexia

The definitive guide to the untapped power of dyslexic thinking and its vital role in our future

by Kate Griggs

Vermilion
LONDON

5

Published in 2021 by Vermilion an imprint of Ebury Publishing,
20 Vauxhall Bridge Road,
London SW1V 2SA

Vermilion is part of the Penguin Random House group of companies
whose addresses can be found at global.penguinrandomhouse.com

Penguin Random House UK

This edition first published by Vermilion in 2021

www.penguin.co.uk

A CIP catalogue record for this book is available from the British Library

ISBN 9781529149265

Printed and bound in Great Britain by Clays Ltd, Elcograf S.p.A.

The authorised representative in the EEA is Penguin Random House Ireland,
Morrison Chambers, 32 Nassau Street, Dublin D02 YH68

FSC www.fsc.org MIX Paper from responsible sources FSC® C018179

Penguin Random House is committed to a sustainable future for our business, our readers and our planet. This book is made from Forest Stewardship Council® certified paper.

Foreword

by Sir Richard Branson

It's official . . . the world needs Dyslexic Thinking.

This is Dyslexia is not only a brilliant guide for people with dyslexia. It also helps parents, employers and educators truly understand dyslexia and Dyslexic Thinking.

It outlines why it's time to redefine dyslexia, to value the massive benefits it can bring and to empower every person with dyslexia to unleash their superpowers.

I simply wouldn't be where I am today if I wasn't dyslexic. In the real world, dyslexia can be a huge advantage. Many people with dyslexia have great imaginations, creativity and problem-solving skills. In fact, many of the world's greatest entrepreneurs and inventors are dyslexic. Thomas Edison's light bulb illuminated our lives, Henry Ford made cars accessible to all and Steve Jobs gave us the iPhone.

Now, post-pandemic, our world is in a period of rapid change. New research by ManpowerGroup Talent Solutions and Made By Dyslexia finds that by 2025, 50 per cent of all jobs will be done by machines and the skills that humans need to set themselves apart and compete in this new hybrid workforce of the future are Dyslexic Thinking skills.

So, whether you're dyslexic or not, it's time to value Dyslexic Thinking and the vital role it can play in all our futures.

That's been one of my mantras – focus and simplicity. Simple can be harder than complex; you have to work hard to get your thinking clean and simple.

Steve Jobs

#MadeByDyslexia

It's imagination, intuition and empathy that sets us apart from the machines. And that's Dyslexic Thinking.

Kate Griggs

#MadeByDyslexia

About this book

This book is packed with everything you need to know about dyslexia, written in a style that people Made By Dyslexia will find easy to absorb.

It is reassuringly short and uses images and infographics where helpful.

Because dyslexics love to see the big picture, there are bullet point summaries at the end of each chapter and information included as lists.

Throughout the book there is a blend of written and digital storytelling. A blend of words, pictures and videos suits the multisensory way dyslexics like to consume information.

What's more Made by Dyslexia has some amazing videos and resources to help you understand dyslexia. Look out for the QR codes throughout the book, which will take you to inspiring videos and must-see interviews.

You can read this book from beginning to end, or dip into any section and jump around to take the information most valuable to you. After all, dyslexics like to do things differently.

Imagine a world where people with dyslexia are educated in a way that supports them. It means anything is possible . . . anything is possible.

Orlando Bloom

#MadeByDyslexia

Contents

PART 1: The Big Picture – Introduction

- *5 reasons why EVERYONE should read this book* 2
- *5 facts about me* 7
- *5 facts about Made By Dyslexia* 12
- *Twenty-first Century Definition of Dyslexia* 15

PART 2: THIS is Dyslexia

- *10 key facts about dyslexia* 18
- *Why dyslexics think differently* 23
- *Dyslexic greats* 33
- *10 key facts about identifying dyslexia* 46
- *Dyslexic Thinking skills explained* 49
    - Visualising 53
    - Imagining 53
    - Communicating 54
    - Reasoning 55
    - Connecting 56
    - Exploring 57
- *The value of Dyslexic Thinking* 60
- *Dyslexic Thinking skills quiz* 65
- *Dyslexic Challenges* 80

PART 3: THIS is Dyslexia in Action
- *Dyslexic intelligence – 5 reasons why dyslexics make top spies* 91
- *5 reasons why dyslexics make powerful change-makers* 98
- *5 reasons why dyslexics make great entrepreneurs* 107
- *5 reasons why dyslexics make skilled communicators* 117
- *5 reasons why dyslexics make great imaginers* 126
- *5 reasons why dyslexics make unstoppable sports champions* 134
- *Dyslexic inventions – 5 of the greatest breakthroughs Made By Dyslexia* 144
- *Dyslexia in the workplace – 5 top tips from our community* 154

PART 4: THIS is Dyslexia in Kids
- *How to spot, support and empower dyslexic children* 165
- *Dyslexic Thinking skills in children explained* 180
- *7 Thinking Skills Archetypes* 182
  - Storytellers 184
  - Makers 184
  - Entertainers 185
  - Movers 186
  - Imaginers 186

- Questioners 187
- 'People' People 188
- *Dyslexic Challenges* 194
- *Growing up Made By Dyslexia – 5 top tips* 202

PART 5: 5 Steps to Change
- *5 ways to make a difference* 209
  - Everyone 209
  - Families 209
  - Kids 209
  - Teachers 209
  - Employers 210
- *5 reasons why we must act NOW* 211

References 214
About the Author 221

We do have to look at things differently, if we're going to combat some of the challenges that every young person is facing for the twenty-first century. The time is now.

HRH Princess Beatrice

#MadeByDyslexia

If we did everything
we are capable of,
we would literally
astound ourselves.

Thomas Edison

#MadeByDyslexia

PART 1:

The Big Picture – Introduction

5 REASONS WHY EVERYONE SHOULD READ THIS BOOK

1. **It's official – the future needs Dyslexic Thinking**
   In 2018[1] and 2019,[2] my charity – Made By Dyslexia – partnered with Ernst & Young (EY) to produce the 'Value of Dyslexia' reports. These groundbreaking reports highlight a crucial fact: in a fast-paced and changing workplace, where machines are poised to take over many tasks, **dyslexics have exactly the skills needed for the workplace of tomorrow**. Our 2021 report with ManpowerGroup found that the pandemic has turbocharged this change and by 2025 humans and machines will split work 50:50.[3] The 50 per cent of human skills are an exact match of Dyslexic Thinking skills. **So, dyslexic or not, you need to understand Dyslexic Thinking and its vital role in all our futures . . . or be left behind!**

2. **The good news – dyslexia is VERY common and there are lots of us!**
   As many as one in five people are dyslexic,[4] that's 20 per cent of the global population,

and over one billion people. That means that in every class and every workplace, all around the world, there are one in five people already hardwired with the skills we need for the future. We just need to make sure we all know how to spot them and how to empower them. **This book will help you do exactly that.**

3. **Redefining dyslexia – for the twenty-first century**
   Dyslexia is largely understood to be a learning difficulty or disability, so it's unsurprising many of us hide it and are embarrassed by it. Dyslexia does come with its challenges in 'traditional' learning and in the tests used to 'benchmark' students and employees. But now those challenges are being mitigated by technology and companies are placing huge value on our strengths (as shown in the diagram on page 62, adapted from the EY report). **This book helps you to see dyslexia as a strength and encourages everyone to harness it.**

4. **Reshaping education – for the twenty-first century**
   Right now, education systems around the world aren't spotting, supporting or empowering dyslexic children. Only 20 per cent of dyslexic students are identified at school,[5] so 80 per

cent are being left to 'muddle through', feeling that school, and them, don't quite fit. Worse still, Made By Dyslexia research found that 91 per cent of teachers have little or no understanding of Dyslexic Strengths.[6] So, despite dyslexics being ready for the workplace of tomorrow, we must reshape how we teach them today. **This book will help everyone spot dyslexia.**

5. **Different times – different measures**
Our fast-changing world is facing unprecedented challenges, so now more than ever, we need minds who think differently to solve the many problems we face and to shape our futures. Without a doubt, we need Dyslexic Thinking. But measuring intelligence, success and eligibility using the same standardised tests and traditional benchmarking that we have used for decades, in education and the workplace, is no longer fit for purpose and is actually filtering out the very types of minds we need. **This book will help you view intelligence differently.**

The Skills of the Future graph (see page 62), adapted from our EY report, clearly shows that technology can now mitigate a lot of Dyslexic Challenges, leaving us free to focus on our strengths. All of the empty circles in the bottom left-hand corner represent Dyslexic Challenges and are the skills that technology and machines are now taking over. The smiley faces in the top right-hand corner reflect our Dyslexic Strengths, which are the skills that machines will not be able to do.

So, with Dyslexic Strengths now in high demand, and our challenges of less importance in this new hybrid world, dyslexics have every reason to smile – because now really is our time to shine!

We're here to put a dent in the universe. Otherwise, why else even be here?

Steve Jobs

#MadeByDyslexia

5 FACTS ABOUT ME

1. **I'm Made By Dyslexia**
   Like me, almost my entire family are dyslexic: my dad, brother, aunts, uncles, nieces, nephews, cousins. I even married a dyslexic (they say like attracts like!) so it's no surprise that both our sons are dyslexic, and their partners too! I've been surrounded by an extraordinary 'smorgasbord' of Dyslexic Thinking for as long as I can remember. Together we've been through a myriad of experiences that have brought me to where I am today: founding and running the global charity, Made By Dyslexia, and writing this book.

2. **I've experienced first-hand what's bad, and what's good**
   Up until I was eight years old, my schooling was a disaster! Looking back at my school reports I was a classic dyslexic, but my first school didn't spot it. Instead, I was a 'must try harder' 'quiet girl' who HATED school because I felt like a failure. When I failed entrance exams aged nine, I was sent to a new school, which was mainstream but one that understood and embraced dyslexia, and

in a matter of weeks my life was totally transformed. This transformation was made possible by teachers who were trained to spot and support us, and who focused on Dyslexic Strengths. It was that simple!

3. **I'm driven by a personal passion to create change**
   My son Ted was a happy-go-lucky, creative little chap . . . until he started school at the age of four. All of my early school nightmares came back to haunt me as the same challenges I had experienced were happening to Ted, but much worse. I was genuinely shocked that 30+ years on his teachers didn't know how to spot and support his obvious dyslexic struggles or his amazing Dyslexic Strengths. So, I had some training in dyslexia so I could help Ted, which was when I realised how common our experiences were. We were lucky to be able to send Ted to my old school (where, like me, he flourished). But, as soon as he was settled, I then set about trying to change things.

4. **I'm a campaigner and researcher**
   I have been campaigning and researching in the field of dyslexia since 2005. My first campaign included a BBC One documentary[7]

and resulted in the UK government conducting an official review of dyslexia.[8] This led to a huge investment in teacher training. I've spent years researching Dyslexic Strengths and in 2017 I set up Made By Dyslexia, a global charity with a mission to help the world properly understand, value and support Dyslexic Thinking. With the help of our celebrity supporters, we are redefining dyslexia. In partnership with forward-thinking companies like EY and ManpowerGroup, we're creating compelling research highlighting the need for change in work and schools. And with Microsoft, we've created free online training; our mission is to train every teacher in the world.

5. **I'm a speaker and an author, hoping to inspire a movement**
   My mission is to help the world understand Dyslexic Strengths and I want to communicate this in any way and wherever I can. I've spoken at events all around the world, including a TEDx Talk, and I published a children's book, *Xtraordinary People*[9], last year, which is the first book to explain Dyslexic Thinking skills in kids; I was beyond excited when it got to number one on Amazon!

When I started my campaigning, no one spoke about Dyslexic Strengths; now we have a growing global social movement of proud, passionate dyslexics and their families pushing for change, all over the world. I am so proud of the part I've played in empowering and energising the extraordinary dyslexic movement and community around the world.

Join us . . . change is coming!

Kate Griggs
2021

As a charity, our goal is not to exist. If we redefine dyslexia, and make sure every teacher and every employer can spot, support and empower every dyslexic, then our job is done!

Kate Griggs

#MadeByDyslexia

5 FACTS ABOUT MADE BY DYSLEXIA

1. Made By Dyslexia is a global charity led by successful dyslexics

> ***Watch*** *our award-winning* 'Made By Dyslexia Sperm Bank Film' *to learn more:*

2. Our purpose is to redefine dyslexia and help the world understand, value and support it

> ***Watch*** *our* 'Value of Dyslexia Report' *film to learn more:*

3. Our goal is to train every teacher in the world with free online training

***Watch** our* 'Connect the Spots' *film to learn more:*

4. Our mission is to help every child understand their Dyslexic Superpowers

***Watch** our* 'Xtraordinary People' *film to learn more:*

5. Our campaign to redefine dyslexia, launches during the UN General Assembly 2021

***Watch** our* 'THIS is Dyslexia' *film to learn more:*

Visit www.madebydyslexia.org for
lots more information.
Join the @madebydyslexia movement on our social channels: Facebook, Twitter, Instagram, LinkedIn.

TWENTY-FIRST CENTURY DEFINITION OF DYSLEXIA

Dyslexia influences as many as one in five people and is a genetic difference in an individual's ability to learn and process information. As a result, dyslexic individuals have differing abilities, with strengths in creative, problem-solving and communication skills but face challenges with spelling, reading and memorising facts. Generally, a dyslexic cognitive profile will be uneven when compared to a neurotypical cognitive profile. This means that dyslexic individuals really do think differently. Traditional benchmarking disadvantages dyslexics, measuring them against the very things they find challenging.

PART 2:

THIS is Dyslexia

10 KEY FACTS ABOUT DYSLEXIA

1. As many as one in five people are dyslexic.[1]
2. Dyslexia is genetic, so it runs in families.
3. Dyslexic brains are 'wired' slightly differently, meaning they have a different way of processing information.
4. This difference results in a pattern of strengths like critical thinking, creativity, emotional intelligence and communication skills.
5. It also results in challenges affecting traditional learning such as reading, writing, spelling, rote learning, memory and concentration.
6. Each dyslexic will have a different pattern of Strengths and Challenges.
7. Identification is key to our success in education and employment as well as our self-esteem.
8. If we place equal importance on Dyslexic Strengths and Challenges, we can and will go far.
9. Four in five successful dyslexics attribute Dyslexic Thinking to their success.[2]

10. Research tells us that Dyslexic Thinking skills are vital for the future.[3]

Watch *celebrities including Orlando Bloom, Sir Richard Branson, Dr Maggie Aderin-Pocock and Keira Knightley tell you more about their dyslexia and why it makes them brilliant at what they do:*

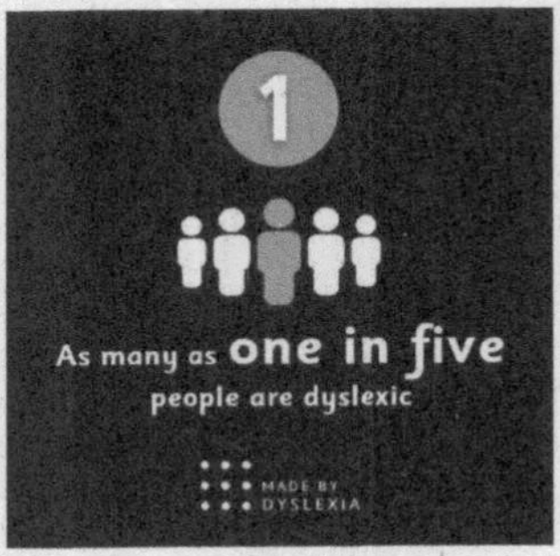
1
As many as one in five
people are dyslexic
MADE BY
DYSLEXIA

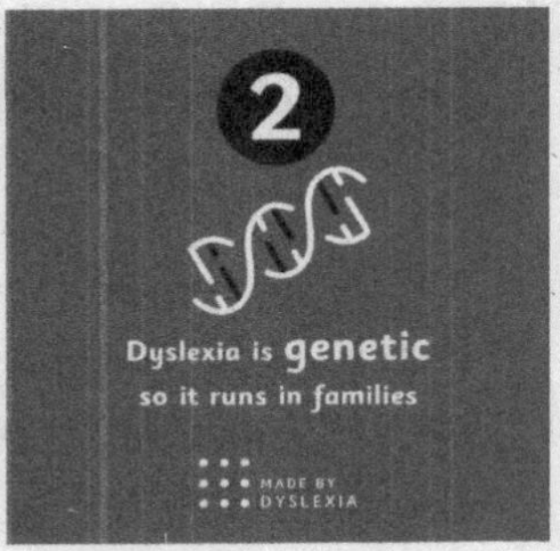
2
Dyslexia is genetic
so it runs in families
MADE BY
DYSLEXIA

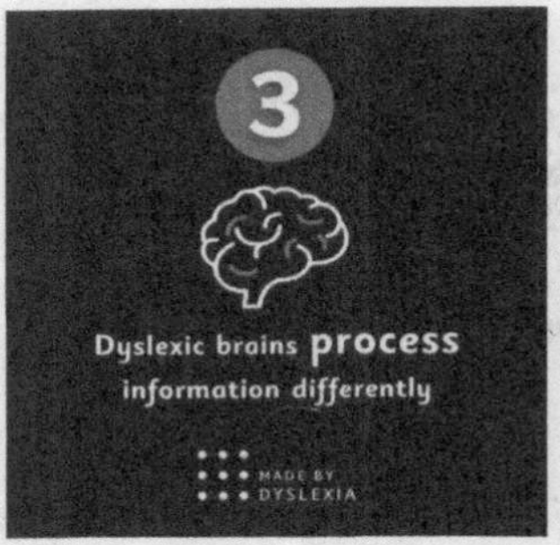
3
Dyslexic brains process
information differently
MADE BY
DYSLEXIA

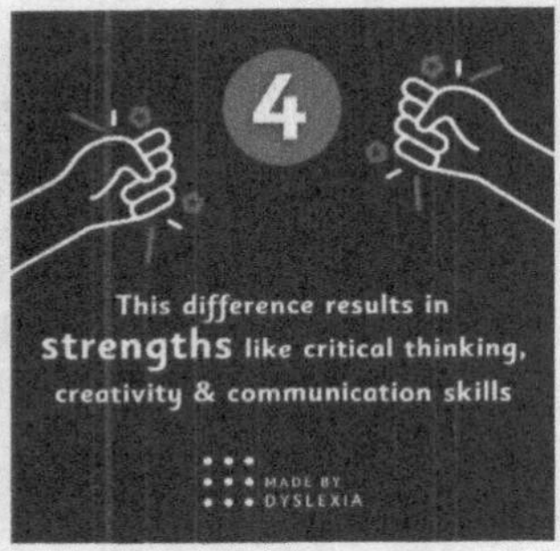
4
This difference results in
strengths like critical thinking,
creativity & communication skills
MADE BY
DYSLEXIA

5
And challenges with reading,
writing, spelling, rote learning,
memory & concentration
MADE BY
DYSLEXIA

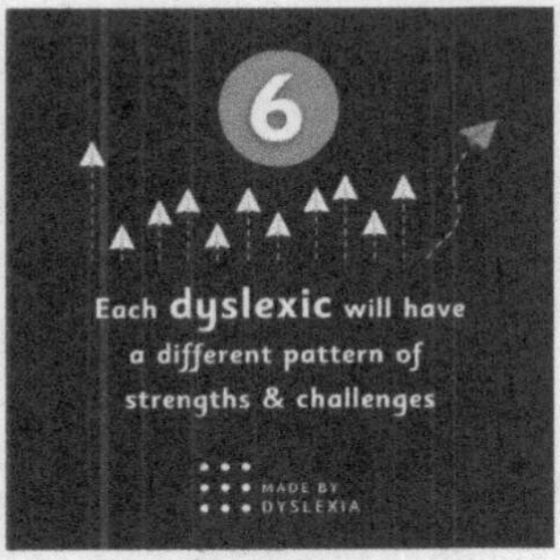
6
Each dyslexic will have
a different pattern of
strengths & challenges
MADE BY
DYSLEXIA

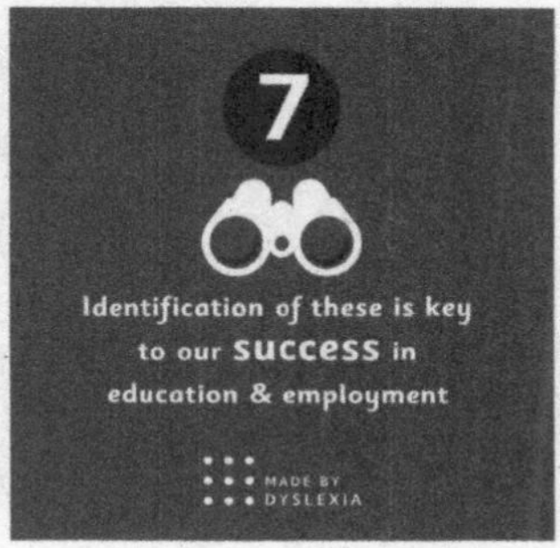
7
Identification of these is key
to our success in
education & employment
MADE BY
DYSLEXIA

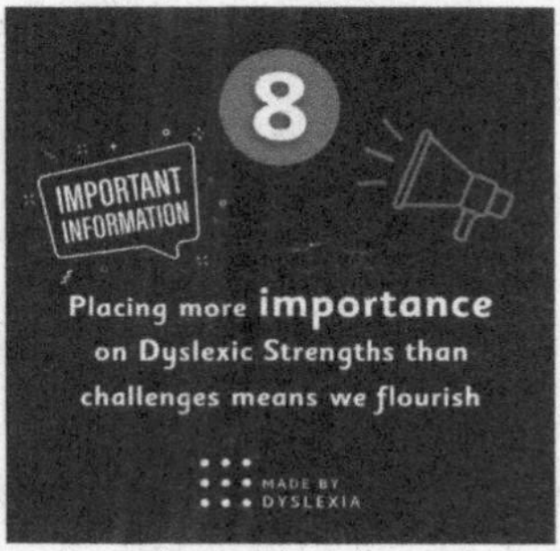
8
IMPORTANT
INFORMATION
Placing more importance
on Dyslexic Strengths than
challenges means we flourish
MADE BY
DYSLEXIA

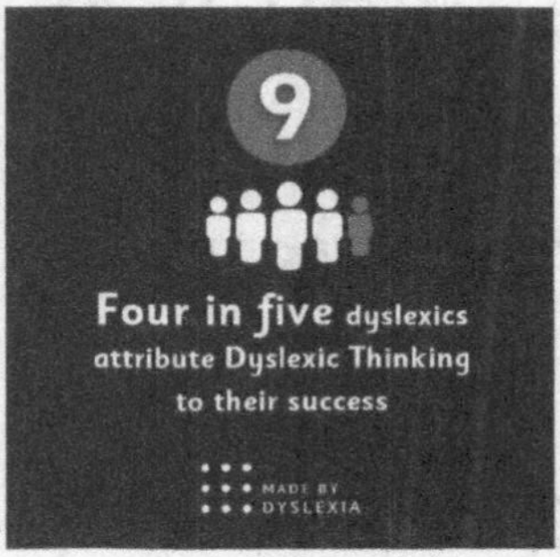
9
Four in five dyslexics
attribute Dyslexic Thinking
to their success
MADE BY
DYSLEXIA

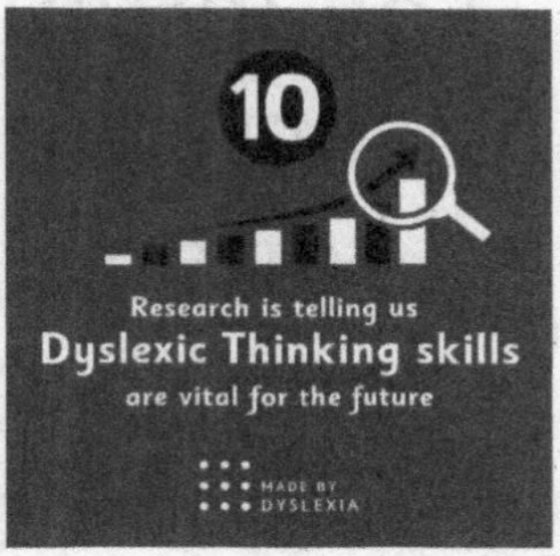
10
Research is telling us
Dyslexic Thinking skills
are vital for the future
MADE BY
DYSLEXIA

The intuitive mind is a sacred gift and the rational mind is a faithful servant. We have created a society that honours the servant and has forgotten the gift.

Albert Einstein

#MadeByDyslexia

WHY DYSLEXICS THINK DIFFERENTLY

Dyslexic minds process information differently. We are naturally curious and highly creative with an ability to unconventionally connect the dots and think laterally. We have strengths in areas like creativity, problem-solving, empathy and communication but face challenges with things like spelling, reading, rote learning and memorising facts. Each dyslexic will have different Strengths and Challenges.

Generally, a dyslexic profile will be uneven (some call it 'spiky') when compared to a neurotypical profile. This simply means we're exceptionally good at some things (often in the top percentiles) and we really struggle with other areas (often in the low percentiles). This means we need a slightly different approach to teaching or work, with small accommodations and technology to help mitigate our challenges.

THE POWER OF DYSLEXIC THINKING

Many dyslexics have amazing abilities to imagine and innovate, and have gone on to transform the world we live in. Famous dyslexics include Thomas

Edison, who illuminated our lives with the light bulb; Steve Jobs, who gave us 'pocket computers' with the iPhone, and Ingvar Kamprad, who founded IKEA and the flat-pack furniture that revolutionised how we shop.

- **We imagine new ideas that jolt society forwards . . .** from the iPhone and motor car, to the first aeroplane and the light bulb.
- **We visualise space differently . . .** making us world-class architects, champion sports stars and F1-winning racing drivers.
- **We're expert storytellers and gifted writers . . .** creating characters and plots that captivate and use language in surprising and refreshingly different ways, from Steven Spielberg to Roald Dahl and Agatha Christie.
- **We're curious learners, asking 'what if?' and 'why not?' . . .** leading us to make scientific breakthroughs, from space travel to stem cells.
- **We're skilled communicators, big-picture thinkers, inspirational leaders and exceptional orators . . .** from Winston Churchill to Sir Richard Branson.
- **We spot patterns, simplify complex info and excel at analysing data . . .** making us

top spies and gifted members of the intelligence service.

ROUND PEGS IN SQUARE HOLES

However, while our Dyslexic Thinking may have changed the world, at school we're likely to feel bottom of the class. That's because the education system isn't designed for Dyslexic Thinking. It is largely about knowledge-based rote learning and high-stakes standardised tests, which need fine-detail processing and great memorisation of facts – areas that are Dyslexic Challenges.

Worse still, most teachers aren't trained to spot, support and value our dyslexic abilities, so for many, we'll go through life without knowing we are dyslexic and never fully understand our extraordinary potential. That can leave many of us feeling that school and 'us' don't quite fit.

And we take that feeling of not quite fitting into our working life too, with around three out of four dyslexics saying they hide their dyslexia from their employers.[4] Many feel they must try to fit in, when actually we should be allowing our amazing Dyslexic Strengths to stand out. Because at work, too, we are faced with standardised tests that don't suit our non-standard, divergent thinking and our strengths are not always fully understood or capitalised upon, either.

But times are changing.

MINDS MADE FOR THE TWENTY-FIRST CENTURY

In 2018[5] and 2019[6] we released two groundbreaking 'Value of Dyslexia' reports with EY. The reports highlight how important Dyslexic Thinking is for the future, finding that as the world of work is automated and AI takes over, many of the jobs of the future will need Dyslexic Thinking skills.

Our 2021 'The Dyslexic Dynamic' report with ManpowerGroup[7] highlights that Dyslexic Thinking skills are even more vital for the post-COVID recovery. The pandemic has sped up the implementation of AI and automation, predicting that by 2025, 50 per cent of jobs will be done by machines, and the remaining 50 per cent of jobs done by the 'human workforce' will require the **exact** skills that dyslexics have.

Matthew Higgs, Global Product Management Director at ManpowerGroup explains:

> ***Last year we saw the biggest workforce shift and reallocation of skills since World War II and today we are seeing the emergence of***

a K-shaped, two-speed recovery. Some industries and people are bouncing back faster and better – those in growth sectors and those with high-demand skills – while others at risk of falling further behind are in urgent need of upskilling and reskilling. It has been inspiring working with Made by Dyslexia to see how dyslexics excel in the human skills that organisations need to complement their digitisation strategies. Soft skills like communications, time management, prioritisation, adaptability, analytical thinking, initiative-taking and empathy are all skills matching the strengths of Dyslexic Thinking and are more highly valued and sought after by employers than ever before. I see it first-hand with my son, Thomas, who is dyslexic and shows so many of the amazing superpowers. I hope that through the work being done by Made by Dyslexia, the education sector and workforce solutions companies such as ManpowerGroup, children like Thomas will be able to enter a more inclusive world of work and organisations will be able to see the full potential of tapping into the dyslexic talent pool to close the skills gap.

So, it's never been more important for everyone to understand and value dyslexia.

THE EMERGENCE OF THE K-SHAPED RECOVERY[8]

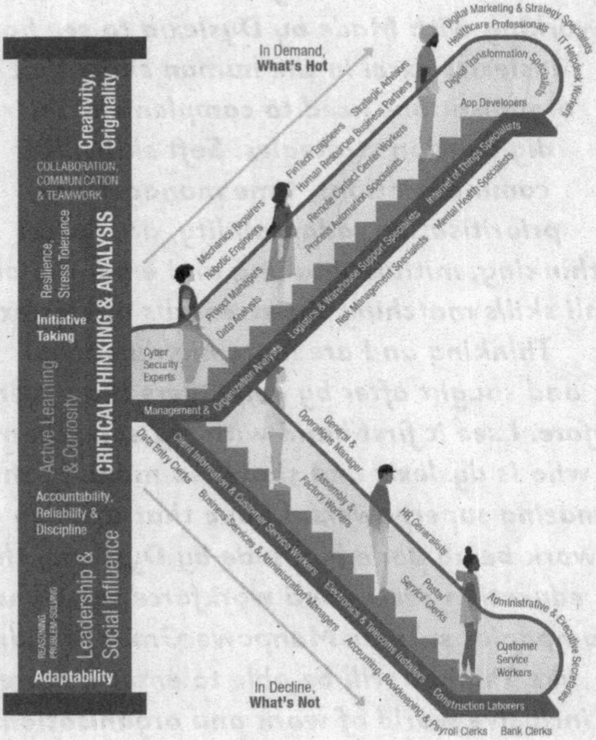

WHAT MAKES DYSLEXICS THINK DIFFERENTLY?

Neuroscience and fMRI scanning of dyslexic brains shows that our brains really are 'wired' differently. The left parietal temporal area of our brains uses different neural pathways that help people with dyslexia to think differently, creatively and laterally.

Dr Manuel Casanova of University of Kentucky School of Medicine[9] studied the connectivity of the brain, specifically the differing length of the axons linking the minicolumns in both dyslexic and non-dyslexic brains, and the significance this has to cognitive reasoning.

WE SEE THE BIG PICTURE

Dr Casanova found that dyslexic brains have a bias to long-distance connections (axons) between minicolumns, which he suggests leads both to the 'big picture processing skill' and a weakness in 'fine-detail processing' that we find in dyslexics. Providing a real-life application to this research, ***nine out of ten*** dyslexics describe their thinking as being able to 'see past detail to gain a strategic (big-picture) view of a subject or problem'. For dyslexics, this can mean that we see the forest, not the trees, or that we have a 'helicopter view' of a situation or problem.

An example of where this type of thinking is a huge advantage in the real world is the Government Communication Headquarters (GCHQ), the British cyber intelligence agency who actively recruit dyslexic people for their ability to think differently. They recognise that they can use their different thinking to solve problems and see patterns that others can't.

You can learn more about the vital role dyslexia plays at GCHQ, and why dyslexics make great spies later in the book. Plus, you can watch our interviews with dyslexic spies and the Director of GCHQ here.

5 Key Points

1. Dyslexics literally think and process information differently.
2. Dyslexia gives you a pattern of strengths like creativity, problem-solving, communication, visualising and much more.
3. Dyslexia comes with challenges such as reading, writing, spelling, rote learning, memory and concentration.
4. Dyslexics have used their strengths to change the world we live in, inventing everything from the iPhone to the light bulb.
5. Dyslexic minds are made for the twenty-first century – they have the exact skills needed for the future workforce.

Some of the greatest breakthroughs in history have come from the dyslexic mind's refusal to accept the status quo.

Josh Clark

#MadeByDyslexia

DYSLEXIC GREATS

There are many examples of extraordinary dyslexic people who have used their Dyslexic Thinking to become great at what they do. Here are our favourites!

5 GREAT DYSLEXIC THINKERS

Albert Einstein – one of the greatest physicists of all time

Steven Hawking – mathematician, physicist and cosmologist

Thomas Edison – the inventor of the light bulb

Henry Ford – the inventor of the motor car

The Wright brothers – the inventors of the aeroplane

5 GREAT DYSLEXIC BRANDS

Apple

IKEA

Virgin

Jo Malone

Soho House

The true sign of intelligence is not knowledge but imagination.

Albert Einstein

#MadeByDyslexia

5 GREAT DYSLEXIC MUSICIANS

John Lennon

Paul McCartney

Michael Bublé

Ed Sheeran

Gwen Stefani

5 GREAT DYSLEXIC FILM DIRECTORS

Steven Spielberg

Steve McQueen

Quentin Tarantino

Guy Ritchie

Spike Lee

5 GREAT DYSLEXIC ACTORS

Will Smith

Keira Knightley

Orlando Bloom

Sir Anthony Hopkins

Whoopi Goldberg

Have the courage
to follow your heart
and intuition.
They somehow know
what you truly
want to become.

Steve Jobs

#MadeByDyslexia

5 GREAT DYSLEXIC SPORTSPEOPLE

Muhammad Ali – one of the greatest heavyweight boxers of all time

Lewis Hamilton – the most successful F1 racing car driver (along with Michael Schumacher)

Sir Jackie Stewart – legendary F1 racing car driver

Kobe Bryant – one of the greatest basketball players of all time

David Beckham – legendary English footballer

5 GREAT DYSLEXIC STORYTELLERS

Agatha Christie – bestselling fiction writer of all time

Roald Dahl – author of *The BFG, The Witches* and more

Ocean Vuong – novelist and poet

Dav Pilkey – creator of *Captain Underpants*

F. Scott Fitzgerald – author of *The Great Gatsby*

You're all geniuses. You don't need anybody to tell you who or what you are.

John Lennon

#MadeByDyslexia

5 GREAT DYSLEXIC DESIGNERS

Tom Ford

Tommy Hilfiger

Victoria Beckham

Alexander McQueen

Sir Paul Smith

All directors are storytellers, so the motivation was to tell the story I wanted to tell. That's what I love.

Spike Lee

#MadeByDyslexia

We're born with success. It is only others who point out our failures, and what they attribute to us as failure.

Whoopi Goldberg

#MadeByDyslexia

It's the repetition of affirmations that leads to belief. And once that belief becomes a deep conviction, things begin to happen.

Muhammad Ali

#MadeByDyslexia

Those who don't believe in magic will never find it.

Roald Dahl

#MadeByDyslexia

We're very curious, we're very inventive, we don't follow the crowd.

Paul Smith

#MadeByDyslexia

Once you know you're dyslexic then school and life take on a whole new dimension.

Dr Maggie Aderin-Pocock

#MadeByDyslexia

10 KEY FACTS ABOUT IDENTIFYING DYSLEXIA

1. Dyslexia can be identified at five years of age or earlier, which is when many dyslexic kids show signs.
2. The earlier it is discovered and supported, the sooner dyslexic kids catch up and keep up.
3. Only one in five dyslexics are identified at school so **80 per cent** leave school unidentified.[10]
4. Dyslexia is not just about learning to read; we can still be proficient readers and dyslexic.
5. A mismatch in what an individual seems capable of and the written work they produce is a strong indicator of dyslexia.
6. The 'label' is vital for our own self-understanding at any age.
7. Unidentified dyslexia can cause low self-esteem in childhood and into adult life.
8. Four in five dyslexics say that knowing they were dyslexic helped them develop the perseverance needed to succeed.[11]

9. Adjustments and accommodations that come with identification are crucial for our success.

10. Traditional tests and teaching mean we often 'fail' despite good knowledge and ability:

   - Nine in 10 dyslexics have poor spelling, punctuation and grammar but are great writers.[12]
   - Seven in 10 struggle to learn times tables but around half of dyslexics are great at maths.[13]
   - Nine in 10 struggle getting their thoughts onto paper.[14]

Watch *our* 'Dyslexia Awareness: Identification' *film:*

TAKE THE TEST

If you think you might be dyslexic, or know someone who is, take our Dyslexic Thinking test at the end of Part 2 or online at www.madebydyslexia.org

My dyslexia is not a disability, but an ability to think differently, and if this world needs anything at this moment, it is people who think differently.

Jo Malone

#MadeByDyslexia

DYSLEXIC THINKING SKILLS EXPLAINED

I have many family members and friends who are dyslexic, and I feel lucky to have been surrounded by Dyslexic Thinking all of my life.

Throughout my time as a campaigner and researcher in the field of dyslexia, I have met and interviewed thousands of successful dyslexics and engaged with experts and leading thinkers on dyslexia from around the globe. Together, we have found that dyslexics really do think differently and, if harnessed, this difference can lead to brilliant careers and fulfilled lives.

But despite everything we know, and decades of success stories, few people actually understand or value Dyslexic Thinking. In fact, when we launched Made By Dyslexia, our research (conducted with YouGov) found that only 3 per cent of people saw dyslexia as an advantage.[15] So, I have made it my life's work to change that.

Dyslexic Thinking skills

Visualising

Interacting with space, senses, physical ideas & new concepts

(75 per cent of dyslexics are above average at visualising)

Imagining

Creating an original piece of work, or giving ideas a new spin

(84 per cent of dyslexics are above average at imagining)

Communicating

Crafting & conveying clear & engaging messages

(71 per cent of dyslexics are above average at communicating)

MADE BY
DYSLEXIA

Reasoning

Understanding patterns, evaluating possibilities & making decisions

(84 per cent of dyslexics are above average at reasoning)

Connecting

Understanding self, connecting, empathising & influencing others

(80 per cent of dyslexics are above average at connecting)

Exploring

Being curious & exploring ideas in a constant & energetic way

(84 per cent of dyslexics are above average at exploring)

DYSLEXIC THINKING UNCOVERED

To define Dyslexic Thinking skills, Made By Dyslexia conducted one of the largest research projects of its kind, assimilating the **latest research** emerging around dyslexic abilities, different intelligences, and the neuroscience that supported it.

We conducted extensive **qualitative research** with dyslexic people, specifically successful dyslexics, gathering unique insight into their strengths, thinking skills, difficulties and the emotional impact of dyslexia.

Plus, we worked with psychologists and psychometricians to identify six key dyslexic skills. Then we carried out **quantitative research,** testing the framework by getting people to rate themselves against the six dyslexic skill areas. The results were then **benchmarked** against a representative group of dyslexic adults.

THIS IS DYSLEXIC THINKING

Visualising – interacting with space, senses, physical ideas and new concepts

Moving: physical interpretation and game playing.
Examples: dancer, musician, sportsperson.

Making: visualising, planning and making.
Examples: engineer, architect, craft worker, programmer, designer, chef, gardener.

Inventing: exploring possibilities, making connections and inventing.
Examples: scientist, technologist, entrepreneur.

When I approach a situation, I like to visualise and imagine the scenario in my head, this has helped me tremendously.

Dr Maggie Aderin-Pocock

Imagining – creating an original piece of work or giving ideas a new spin

Creating: creating completely original work from your imagination.
Examples: designer, artist, composer, writer.

Interpreting: using imagination to give ideas a new twist or fresh angle.
Examples: actor, advertiser, PR, director, photographer.

One of the amazing things about dyslexics is our imagination. I started dreaming from a young age and then began to put those dreams into reality.

Sir Richard Branson

We're very curious, we're very inventive, we don't follow the crowd.

Sir Paul Smith

Communicating – crafting and conveying clear and engaging messages

Explaining: assessing situations/information and explaining to others.
Examples: journalist, marketeer, politician, teacher, campaigner.

Storytelling: creating vivid, engaging experiences in words, pictures and other media.
Examples: writer, games designer, filmmaker, songwriter.

Generally, TV news is an amazing place to trust your dyslexic instincts. You have to look at the big picture, identify the story, tell the story and create a narrative that's simplified, so that an audience can understand the main issues.

Robyn Curnow

As a scientist, I found that I am able to take complex ideas and simplify them, storytell and bring science to life in my own unique way; this has been a huge advantage.

Dr Maggie Aderin-Pocock

Reasoning – understanding patterns, evaluating possibilities and making decisions

Simplifying: understanding, taking apart and simplifying complex ideas and concepts.

Analysing: using logic to decide on the strength of an argument or where the truth lies.

Deciding: interpreting patterns and situations to predict future events and make decisions.

Visioning: seeing past detail to gain a strategic (big-picture) view of a subject or problem.

GCHQ has 100 years of keeping the country safe. When I look at the things ordinary people have done that have ended up with extraordinary outcomes, then I can see people who think differently, and I can see dyslexics in every one of those from 1919 through to the present day.

Jeremy Fleming

It's like a superpower in a way, because you can see things that other people can't.

Leo, Student

Connecting – understanding self, connecting, empathising and influencing others

Understanding self: recognising and managing one's own feelings and understanding how they affect one's own behaviour and that of others.

Understanding others: understanding and interpreting the verbal, physical and emotional reactions of other people.

Influencing: managing, influencing and inspiring constructive emotions in other people.

Empathising: sensing, understanding and responding to how people feel.

Dyslexia gives you the ability to listen and to empathise with people. To not only hear what people are saying, but to get behind what they're saying and to better understand what is going on. The other wonderful thing it gives you is the ability not only to listen, but to talk to people and to explain things, and to empathise with them.

The Rt Revd, Sarah Mullally

Exploring – being curious and exploring ideas in a constant and energetic way

Learning: having a curiosity for finding out new things and learning new skills.

Digging: looking into things in a way that means most is learnt or discovered.

Energising: being so passionate about something it gives a buzz, having a tenacity to learn about it.

Doing: using new knowledge to achieve a result that surprises and pleases one's self or others.

Remember to look up at the stars and not down at your feet. Try to make sense of what you see and wonder about what makes the universe exist. Be curious.

Stephen Hawking

If you are interested in something, no matter what it is, go at it full speed. Embrace it with both arms, hug it, love it and above all become passionate about it.

Roald Dahl

We can always kind of be average and do what's normal. I'm not in this to do what's normal.

Kobe Bryant

#MadeByDyslexia

THE VALUE OF DYSLEXIC THINKING

Dyslexic Thinking skills haven't just shaped our past. They are 'mission critical' to our future, too.

In 2018, we asked EY to help us research the overlap between Dyslexic Thinking skills and the skills of the future, as outlined by the World Economic Forum (WEF). They produced two Value of Dyslexia reports one in 2018[16] and 2019[17] which found that Dyslexic Thinking skills were an **exact** match for the WEF skills of the future. And the skills that were in decline (and would be automated or taken over by machines) were the very skills that dyslexics find challenging.

It was official – organisations need dyslexic thinkers – and those who think like them.

This is explained in the following graph on page 62, adapted from our EY report.[18] It shows that Dyslexic Thinking skills (depicted by smiley faces in the top right-hand corner) are the in-demand skills for the future, according to the WEF, while the skills that are more challenging for dyslexics are in decline (shown as empty circles in the bottom left).

So, there has never been a better time to be Made By Dyslexia.

SKILLS OF THE FUTURE

Useful links:

Take the Dyslexic Thinking test at www.madebydyslexia.org

Watch *our* 'Value of Dyslexia Report' *film to understand the value of Dyslexic Thinking:*

Read the reports at www.madebydyslexia.org

Watch *our* 'Dyslexia Awareness: Dyslexia Strengths' *film:*

Trending and declining competency demand and typical dyslexic capability association, all industries, 2022

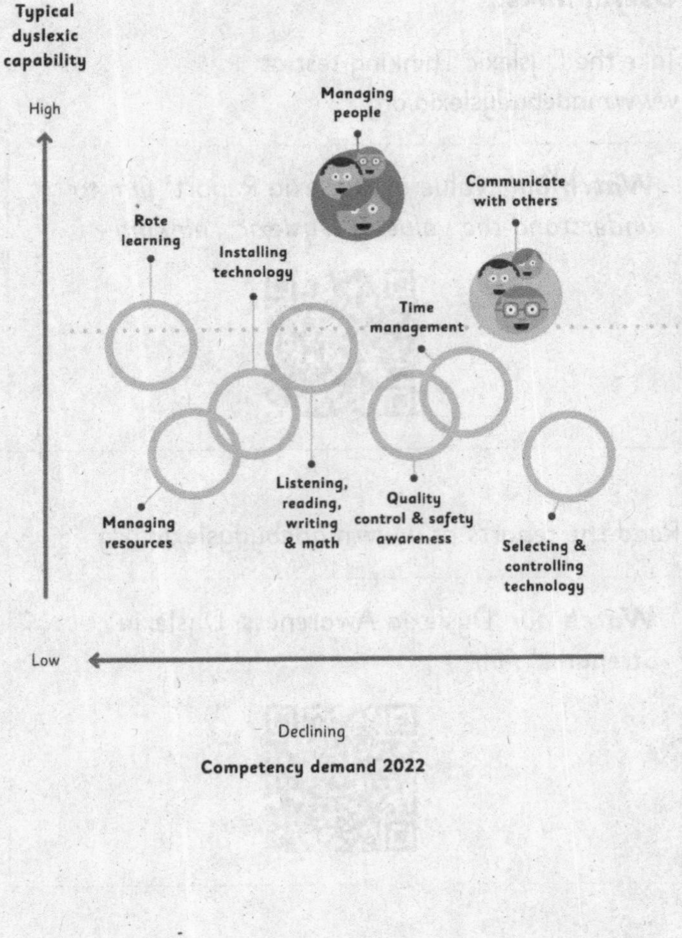

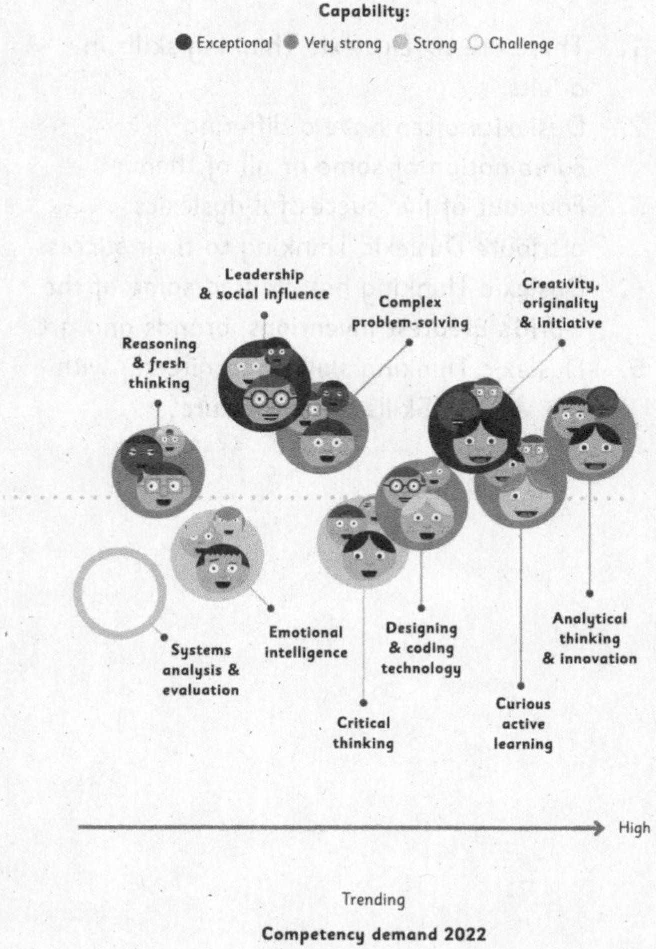
Capability:
Exceptional
Very strong
Strong
Challenge
Leadership & social influence
Complex problem-solving
Creativity, originality & initiative
Reasoning & fresh thinking
Systems analysis & evaluation
Emotional intelligence
Designing & coding technology
Analytical thinking & innovation
Critical thinking
Curious active learning
High
Trending
Competency demand 2022

5 Key Points

1. There are six Dyslexic Thinking skills in adults.
2. Dyslexics often have a differing combination of some or all of them.
3. Four out of five successful dyslexics attribute Dyslexic Thinking to their success.
4. Dyslexic Thinking has created some of the world's greatest inventions, brands and art.
5. Dyslexic Thinking skills map directly with the WEF's 'Skills for the Future'.

DYSLEXIC THINKING SKILLS QUIZ

What are your Dyslexic Thinking skills? And where do your Dyslexic Strengths give you an added advantage? Take our Dyslexic Thinking skills quiz and see. I've shared my results at the end of this quiz.

What's more, if you take this online, you can see a personalised pie chart of your strengths and find out what your top Dyslexic Strength is.
Visit www.madebydyslexia.org

1. VISUALISING

Interacting with space, senses, physical ideas and new concepts.

How good are you at the following? (Select one answer for each question.)

Moving

Using physical interpretation and game playing (like dancers, musicians or sportspeople).

- ❍ Poor
- ❍ Average
- ❍ Good
- ❍ Very Good
- ❍ Excellent

Making

Visualising, planning and making (like engineers, architects, craft workers, programmers, designers, chefs or gardeners).

- ❍ Poor
- ❍ Average
- ❍ Good
- ❍ Very Good
- ❍ Excellent

Inventing

Exploring new possibilities, making connections and inventing new things (like scientists, technologists or entrepreneurs).

- ❍ Poor
- ❍ Average
- ❍ Good
- ❍ Very Good
- ❍ Excellent

2. IMAGINING

Creating an original piece of work, or giving ideas a new spin.

How good are you at the following? (Select one answer for each question.)

Creating

Creating completely original work from your imagination (like designers, artists, composers or writers).

- ❍ Poor
- ❍ Average
- ❍ Good
- ❍ Very Good
- ❍ Excellent

Interpreting

Using your imagination to give ideas a new twist, or bring out a fresh angle (like actors, advertisers, PR people, directors or photographers).

❍ Poor

❍ Average

❍ Good

❍ Very Good

❍ Excellent

3. COMMUNICATION

Crafting and conveying clear and engaging messages.

How good are you at the following? (Select one answer for each question.)

Explaining

Assessing new information or situations and explaining them clearly to other people (like campaigners, journalists, marketeers, politicians or teachers).

- ❍ Poor
- ❍ Average
- ❍ Good
- ❍ Very Good
- ❍ Excellent

Storytelling

Creating vivid and engaging experiences in words, pictures or other media (like authors, writers, games developers, songwriters or filmmakers).

- ❍ Poor
- ❍ Average
- ❍ Good
- ❍ Very Good
- ❍ Excellent

4. REASONING

Understanding patterns, evaluating possibilities and making decisions.

How good are you at the following? (Select one answer for each question.)

Simplifying

Understanding, taking apart and simplifying complex ideas and concepts.

- ❍ Poor
- ❍ Average
- ❍ Good
- ❍ Very Good
- ❍ Excellent

Analysing

Using logic to decide on the strength of an argument or where the truth lies.

- ❍ Poor
- ❍ Average
- ❍ Good
- ❍ Very Good
- ❍ Excellent

Deciding

Interpreting patterns and situations to predict future events and make decisions.

- ❍ Poor
- ❍ Average
- ❍ Good
- ❍ Very Good
- ❍ Excellent

Visioning

Seeing past detail to gain a strategic (big-picture) view of a subject or problem.

- ❍ Poor
- ❍ Average
- ❍ Good
- ❍ Very Good
- ❍ Excellent

5. CONNECTING

Understanding self, connecting, empathising and influencing others.

How good are you at the following? (Select one answer for each question.)

Understanding self

Recognising and managing your own feelings and understanding how they affect your own behaviour and that of others.

❍ Poor

❍ Average

❍ Good

❍ Very Good

❍ Excellent

Understanding others

Understanding and interpreting the verbal, physical and emotional reactions of other people.

❍ Poor

❍ Average

❍ Good

❍ Very Good

❍ Excellent

Influencing

Managing, influencing and inspiring constructive emotions in other people.

- ❍ Poor
- ❍ Average
- ❍ Good
- ❍ Very Good
- ❍ Excellent

Empathising

Sensing, understanding and responding (emotionally and/or practically) to how other people feel.

- ❍ Poor
- ❍ Average
- ❍ Good
- ❍ Very Good
- ❍ Excellent

6. EXPLORING

Being curious and exploring new ideas in a constant and energetic way.

How good are you at the following? (Select one answer for each question.)

Learning

Having great curiosity for finding out new things and learning new skills.

- ❍ Poor
- ❍ Average
- ❍ Good
- ❍ Very Good
- ❍ Excellent

Digging

Looking into things in a way that means that the maximum is learnt or discovered about it.

- ❍ Poor
- ❍ Average
- ❍ Good

- ❍ Very Good
- ❍ Excellent

Energising

Being so passionate about something that it gives a buzz and tenacity to learn about it.

- ❍ Poor
- ❍ Average
- ❍ Good
- ❍ Very Good
- ❍ Excellent

Doing

Jumping in and using new knowledge to achieve a result that surprises and pleases yourself or others.

- ❍ Poor
- ❍ Average
- ❍ Good
- ❍ Very Good
- ❍ Excellent

How did you score? Do your Dyslexic Strengths lie in Connecting or Exploring? Reasoning or Imagining? Are you stronger in Communicating or Visualising? These six skills are what dyslexic minds excel at. Many of us have a mixture of these skills and they're what help us bring a unique and valuable perspective to any team we're part of.

For a personalised chart of your strengths (you will find an example of mine on the next page), visit www.madebydyslexia.org where you can also take a quick test to see if you are dyslexic based on Dyslexic Challenges too.

Your results explained

Your specific skills

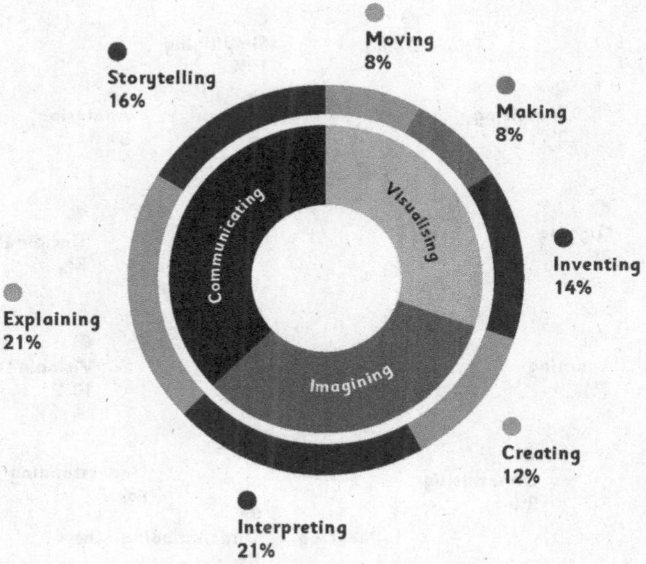

Visualising		**Imagining**		**Communicating**	
Moving	8%	Creating	12%	Explaining	21%
Making	8%	Interpreting	21%	Storytelling	16%
Inventing	14%				

Your results explained

Your general skills

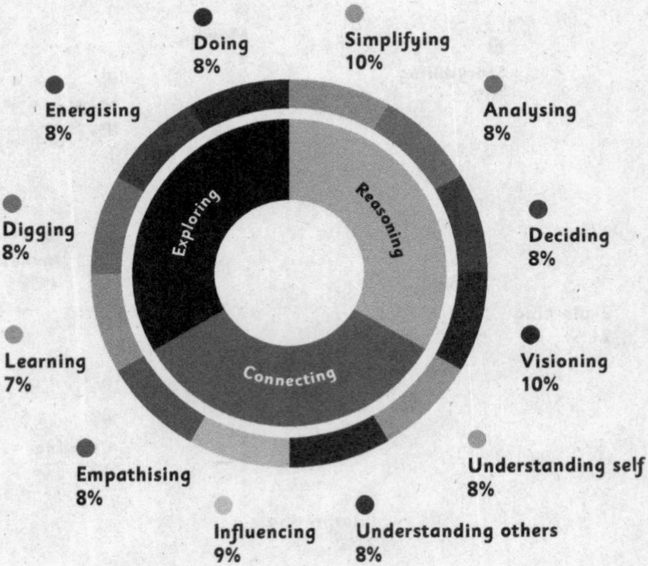

Reasoning		**Connecting**		**Exploring**	
Simplifying	8%	Understanding self	8%	Learning	21%
Analysing	8%	Understanding others	8%	Digging	16%
Deciding	8%	Influencing	8%	Energising	8%
Visioning	8%	Empathising	8%	Doing	8%

My spelling makes people laugh but I was lucky to have a teacher who focused on what I was writing, not how I was spelling it. That let me explore my creativity.

Keira Knightley

#MadeByDyslexia

DYSLEXIC CHALLENGES

THE CHALLENGE OF THINKING DIFFERENTLY

Because our brains process information differently, we sometimes struggle with certain things that others may find easy. These things are often the skills that we are assessed and benchmarked against, or which people generally link to intelligence.

This can make us feel as if we're not as smart as others, which can make others think that too. For example, 89 per cent of dyslexics struggle with spelling and grammar.[19] When a spelling or grammar mistake is made, others are all too quick to pick us up on it and call us out for carelessness, for not checking our work. So, it's hardly surprising that three out of four dyslexics hide their dyslexia from their employers.[20]

CHALLENGING PERCEPTIONS

This is why it's important for everyone to understand Dyslexic Challenges, and to understand that our mistakes are not because we're careless or stupid: they're because we are Made By Dyslexia and have a different way of thinking and processing information.

It's important to remember that if intelligence was measured as the ability to see the big picture or demonstrate creativity, innovation, imagination or communication skills, then dyslexics would ace every exam or work project!

So, when it comes to our challenges, don't be embarrassed to admit that you have them. Be upfront and help others to understand them.

At Made By Dyslexia, we've created a range of assets to help you tell the world that you're Made By Dyslexia. You can add Dyslexic Thinking to your list of skills on LinkedIn or include it on your CV.

You can add a line to your email signature, or to your social profiles that highlights your Dyslexic Strengths and Challenges. Many trailblazing, creative leaders around the world are already using them. Here are some of our favourites:

- I'm #MadeByDyslexia – expect creative thinking and creative spelling.
- I'm #MadeByDyslexia – expect big thinking and small typos.
- I'm #MadeByDyslexia – expect curious ideas and curious spelling.
- I'm #MadeByDyslexia – I'm a quick thinker (sometimes my spelling can't keep up).

You can find out more at www.madebydyslexia.org

HUMOUR CAN HELP

It's really important to have a sense of humour about our challenges, just as Keira Knightley says on page 79. Because, while spellcheckers can be our best friend, there are words that it just won't pick up. For example, one of my recurring mistakes is '*definitely*', which my spellcheck often autocorrects to '*defiantly*', which, of course, will completely change the meaning of what I write!

A member of our team told us a wonderful story about when they were doing some work with Sandra Bullock, and spellcheck didn't pick up the fact that they had put an 'O' in the surname instead of 'U'! Sometimes we need to ask Siri or Alexa to double-check a spelling.

The good thing is, technology can mitigate a lot of our challenges leaving us free to focus on our Dyslexic Strengths, just as the graph earlier (see page 62) shows.

SO, WHAT ARE DYSLEXIC CHALLENGES?

All dyslexics will struggle with some of the following, and these solutions will help.

Reading: Difficulties recognising and manipulating sounds, letters and words, making learning to read difficult. Once we've learnt to read, dyslexics will still remain slow readers.

Solution: *Structured, multisensory phonics programmes will enable every dyslexic to learn to read. Extra time in exams and for assignments, plus seeing notes ahead of time make the world of difference. Using devices and assistive technology, like speech-to-text and text-to-speech can help.*

Memory systems: Challenges with verbal (remembering spoken instructions), sequential (ordering facts and information), working (keeping facts in mind and manipulating them) and visual (recognising symbols, letters and words) memory make rote learning and getting thoughts down quite difficult.

Solution: *Many dyslexic minds find organisers/ planners, mind maps and assistive technology incredibly useful.*

Spelling, punctuation and grammar: To be good at spelling, punctuation and grammar you have to learn and memorise a series of information, skills and rules. Challenges with memory systems make it difficult for dyslexics to learn and apply these rules.

Solution: *Our teachers, managers and peers should be encouraged to focus on the content of what we write, not the spelling, punctuation and grammar. We can use assistive technology like* *spellcheck – Siri, Alexa, Grammarly – and the built-in tools that come with word-processing software and other technology.*

Maths: Challenges with sequential and working memory cause difficulties with times tables and mental maths, although dyslexics are often good at conceptual, high-level maths. So, we often know the answer but cannot tell you how we got there, which is usually required in tests.

Solution: *Look for high-level skills and the ability to 'see the big picture' and jump to the solution. Encourage a love of maths, give support for challenges. Use assistive technology.*

Traditional benchmarks: Standardised tests, high-stakes exams in education and many psychometric tests used in recruitment disadvantage dyslexics because of all the above.

Solution: *Adjustments and extra time in tests and assignments, project work, exploring different testing methods, using assistive technology and video presentations all enable dyslexics to demonstrate their real knowledge and skills in order to thrive.*

SOUND FAMILIAR?

If you recognise these challenges and think you might be dyslexic, or know someone who is, take the Dyslexic Thinking test at the end of Part 2 or online at www.madebydyslexia.org

Useful links:

Watch *our* 'Dyslexia Awareness: Dyslexic Challenges' *film:*

Find a range of ideas and things you can use at www.madebydyslexia.org.

5 Key Points

1. There are five key Dyslexic Challenges: reading; memory systems; spelling, punctuation and grammar; maths; and traditional benchmarks.
2. Dyslexia is a difference in how our minds process information. Find your favourite way to absorb and give information. And tell others that that's how YOU think.
3. Help teachers, managers and peers understand your Dyslexic Strengths and Challenges. If you're at work, try updating your email signature to celebrate your different way of thinking can help.
4. Technology can be transformative in helping dyslexics manage their challenges.
5. Four in five dyslexics say knowing they were dyslexic helped them understand their Strengths and Challenges to succeed. So, it's important to share that you are dyslexic with others.

PART 3:

THIS is Dyslexia in Action

Dyslexia makes,
fights and inspires.
Dyslexia writes and
rewrites everything.
Dyslexia makes history
and the future.

Sir Richard Branson

#MadeByDyslexia

DYSLEXIA IN ACTION

Dyslexic Thinking has transformed the world we live in. Seeing things differently has helped dyslexics to invent things we can't live without, imagine what others couldn't see and solve problems that others couldn't crack.

For over 100 years, the intelligence services has valued the skills and abilities of dyslexic minds. As Jeremy Fleming of GCHQ explains, many of our most important intelligence breakthroughs have come from a dyslexic's ability to solve the seemingly unsolvable.

So . . . in this section we take a closer look at dyslexia in action.

First, we look at the extraordinary role dyslexia has played in the intelligence services, with **5 reasons why dyslexics make top spies**. We explain why our brains are the perfect fit for the intelligence services.

Then we explore **5 of the greatest inventions** of our time and explain how Dyslexic Thinking enabled them to come to be.

Finally, we list ***5 Top Tips*** from the dyslexic people in the global Made By Dyslexia community on what has helped them to thrive.

Before we begin, let's look at **5 areas where dyslexics thrive**, which we will explain why later on.

5 areas where dyslexics thrive

- We make powerful change-makers
- We make great entrepreneurs
- We make skilled communicators
- We make great imaginers
- We make unstoppable sports champions

You'll find real-life stories that are highlighted with quotes, anecdotes or films, which will give you a real sense of **Dyslexia in Action**. Happy exploring!

DYSLEXIC INTELLIGENCE – 5 REASONS WHY DYSLEXICS MAKE TOP SPIES

Here is a little-known fact: Britain's digital intelligence agency, GCHQ actively recruits for dyslexic thinkers, based on their unique skill set.

The impact of dyslexia on keeping us safe as a nation is rarely discussed, but the value of Dyslexic Thinking has been understood by the intelligence community for well over 100 years.

According to Jo Cavan, a senior GCHQ director:

> ***Members of GCHQ's apprenticeship scheme are up to four times more likely than average to be dyslexic.***

The head of GCHQ, Jeremy Fleming, explains:

> ***We see the impact of nation states and terror groups using technology to achieve their harmful agenda. And tackling these challenges requires people who can connect ideas, think visually and use their intuition.***

These are qualities we see a lot of in our dyslexic colleagues.

So, what makes dyslexic minds 'mission critical' to protecting our nation's security?

Here are five reasons why dyslexics make brilliant spies:

1. We see the big picture – the Dyslexic Thinking skill of Reasoning

Dyslexic brains are 'wired' differently. The left parietal temporal area of our brains uses different neural pathways. We are naturally good at Reasoning skills which make us adept at stepping back from the detail and seeing the big picture.

> ***Watch*** *Louise, a secret agent, explain how her dyslexia helps her to see the bigger picture when she's working on a mission:*

2. We can spot patterns others can't – the Dyslexic Thinking skill of Reasoning

While dyslexics may struggle with skills like spelling, punctuation and grammar, they are experts at seeing patterns that others can't. This could be a pattern of behaviour, communication or way to crack a code.

In the D.Spot vodcast, Charlotte (not her real name), an intelligence analyst working in GCHQ's 24/7 operations centre, explained:

I'm often looking through a lot of data and I find that my dyslexia helps me to see the bigger picture and spot patterns that aren't always obvious to everyone else around me. I also find that my approach to finding solutions is very different.

It is no surprise that the most famous codebreaker in Britain, Alan Turing, was believed to have been Made By Dyslexia. Turing was voted in a recent BBC public poll as the greatest person of the twentieth century. As a cryptanalyst based at Bletchley Park during World War II, he broke the Nazis' Enigma code because of his ability to see things from various three-dimensional viewpoints, discern patterns and solve near-impossible problems. Today, many more dyslexic analysts use their Reasoning skills to encrypt systems to keep our nation safe or detect and dismantle systems that seek to do our country harm.

3. We use our intuition to connect the dots – the Dyslexic Thinking skill of Reasoning

Dyslexics often talk about having sudden leaps of insight that help them solve problems in an unconventional way. We use our intuition, and while it may look like daydreaming to others, it is actually our brains thinking around a problem and connecting the dots of insight.

Solving problems creatively and using lateral thinking is a crucial requirement for many of the workforce at GCHQ. Beth Sizeland at GCHQ says:

We've got thousands of examples where dyslexia has given us the critical edge in problem solving.

When the threats come thick and fast from hostile governments, terrorist groups and state-controlled hacktivists, the stakes in solving those problems couldn't be higher.

4. We are gifted analysts – the Dyslexic Thinking skill of Reasoning

The dyslexic mind is extraordinarily good at sifting through large amounts of information, and picking out the key parts.

Jeremy Fleming explains:

Across all of our missions, we have people who are dyslexic, and play a vital role in keeping the country safe . . . I have everyone from the country's best

mathematicians to our most talented engineers and our best analysts, and I can see dyslexics among every one of those.

***Watch** Jeremy explain the value of Dyslexic Thinking to the intelligence world in this interview with Made By Dyslexia:*

5. We are brilliant at simplifying – the Dyslexic Thinking skill of Reasoning

People who are Made By Dyslexia are adept at understanding, taking apart and simplifying complex ideas. This might involve simplifying huge data systems, vast amounts of complex information or picking out a digital trail from millions of imprints online.

THE POWER OF THINKING DIFFERENTLY

Dyslexics are masters of looking at a problem and coming up with an innovative and creative solution.

Rob (not his real name) is an active dyslexic spy at GCHQ who describes his role as a 'transformational innovator'. He works closely with Britain's armed forces and explains:

> ***I use my dyslexic skills to spot opportunities to do things differently. I speak to a lot of people internally who invent stuff and a lot of contacts in the industry and explore how we could use our capabilities in ways that we'd never planned, often to deliver amazing effects.***

It's undoubted that the Dyslexic Strengths of seeing the big picture, spotting patterns, using your intuition to solve impenetrable digital puzzles, simplifying complex information and analysing data all mean that dyslexics are an invaluable part of the mix when it comes to our intelligence service and as Jeremy Fleming says:

> ***We're only going to be successful if we make the most of those who see things differently. Our dyslexic and neurodiverse colleagues are mission critical to GCHQ.***

There's much the rest of the world can learn from this mindset. All of society benefits by harnessing the power of thinking differently.

***Watch** dyslexic spies, Charlotte and Rob, explain why being Made By Dyslexia gives them an added advantage in the covert world of British Intelligence. Tune in to this eye-opening episode of our D.Spot vodcast here:*

Key Points

1. Dyslexic minds are 'mission critical' to protecting our nation's security.
2. Our ability to connect the dots and see the big picture make us extraordinary spies.
3. Dyslexic minds can spot patterns that others can't e.g. behaviour, codes or data.
4. We're brilliant at simplifying processes and coming up with innovative solutions.
5. Spies on GCHQ's apprenticeship scheme are up to **four times** more likely than average to be dyslexic.

5 REASONS WHY DYSLEXICS MAKE POWERFUL CHANGE-MAKERS

What do Winston Churchill, George Washington and HRH Princess Beatrice have in common? They were all Made By Dyslexia. Throughout history, dyslexics have used their strengths to change the world for the better. But what makes dyslexics such powerful makers of change?

Here are five good reasons why dyslexics make powerful change-makers:

1. Dyslexics think big – the Dyslexic Thinking skill of Reasoning

We are driven by a desire to make the world better, fairer. This makes us fearless campaigners with big ambitions. Fierce champions of social mobility. Our Reasoning skills allow us to see past the detail and gain a strategic big-picture view of a situation or problem.

This leads us into careers as campaigners (like me), politicians (eight presidents of the United States are reportedly Made By Dyslexia, including Washington, Eisenhower and Wilson) and into positions that work for social justice. The current CEO of The Prince's Trust and former Chair of the Social Mobility Commission in the UK, Dame Martina Milburn, is proud to be Made By Dyslexia.

***Watch** Dame Martina take part in the Changemakers panel, at the Made By Dyslexia Global Summit:*

2. We're not afraid to challenge the status quo – the Dyslexic Thinking skill of Reasoning

Dyslexics are not content to accept how the world is. Instead, we use our Visioning strengths to imagine how it could be. This allows us to transform whatever field we put our mind to.

Our Exploring strengths mean we ask questions, like 'what if?' and 'why not?', positively disrupting the status quo.

In other areas, we use our courage, persistence and determination to change something and right a wrong. What helps us along the way is our high levels of emotional intelligence and empathy, the sense of wanting to help people. We are often motivated by a strong sense of social justice and equality.

Inspirational activist, Erin Brockovich (a single mum and file clerk secretary at an American law firm) used her Dyslexic Strengths to take on the might of a utility company, whose use of carcinogenic chemicals were poisoning residents of nearby town, Hinkley, California. Even when she was told to drop the case, her determination to challenge the status quo and right a wrong drove her to persist and win a settlement of $333 million for more than 600 residents. It was the largest direct-action lawsuit in US history. She went on to become an environmental activist and continues to fight cases worldwide.

Watch *Erin Brockovich tell her powerful story here:*

Or watch the movie, Erin Brockovich, *where she is brilliantly played by Julia Roberts.*

3. Dyslexics are innovative problem-solvers – the Dyslexic Thinking skill of Reasoning

As dyslexics, our brains process information in a different way. This helps us to come up with new approaches to old problems – an advantage in any workplace. HRH Princess Beatrice says:

One of the strengths we have as dyslexics is to look at things differently, to be a problem-solver, to find new ways to do things.

Our Dyslexic Strengths of Reasoning allow us to understand patterns, evaluate possibilities and make decisions.

Andrew Pike OBE, former Director of the National Security Communication team, explains how he uses his Dyslexic Strengths to his advantage:

I have an unconventional route to problem-solving and find alternative and creative ways to figure things out. I've learnt to play to my dyslexic strengths.

Watch *the Made By Dyslexia interview with HRH Princess Beatrice here:*

4. Dyslexics are great communicators and storytellers – the Dyslexic Thinking skill of Communicating

We act in bold ways that get us noticed and allow our messages to cut through. We think creatively and laterally. And we're able to create a compelling narrative around an issue that helps people understand it and realise it's time for change.

When I launched Made By Dyslexia in 2017, I did it by claiming to open the world's first-ever 'Dyslexic Sperm Bank': a great launch stunt which allowed us to get across our message that dyslexia comes with so many gifts and strengths that can bring you success in life, rather than hold you back. It was a powerful piece of storytelling, watched by 70 million people in just three days.

I've spoken about the creative brilliance of dyslexia in my TEDx Talk too.[1] For me, it's all part of the creative edge dyslexia can give you.

Watch *my TEDx Talk here:*

Dyslexic minds are brilliant at exploring, too. Our curiosity means we find out all there is to know on a topic and use our passion to share it, thereby inspiring change.

My own research into Dyslexic Strengths led me to start Made By Dyslexia. And to partner with Microsoft to create free online 'Dyslexia Awareness' training.

Watch *our* 'Dyslexia Awareness' *training films here:*

5. We are masters in overcoming adversity – the Dyslexic Thinking Skill of Imagining

Finally, dyslexics are resilient. We don't see problems, we see possibilities – springboards that help us achieve what we need to do. Tenacious and driven, we think laterally to solve problems.

Jo Malone says:

> ***My dyslexia means I've learnt how to see around walls, climb ladders and spot the potential in something that others don't.***

This drives us to make the impossible, possible. To find new and different ways to solve things. And to never take no for an answer . . .

Erin Brockovich talks about what her mother used to call 'stick-to-it-ness':

> ***I was a dyslexic. Every time I came home from school with another 'D' stamped on a test and feeling defeated, my mom would say: 'You have to buck up Erin, where's your stick-to-it-ness'. And that struck a chord. Even today, when I hit that wall, I hear my mother. Stick-to-it-ness. It's that persistence. It's that obligation, that stubbornness and you can rise . . . and you can do it.***

At Made By Dyslexia, we're shaped by a certain kind of stick-to-it-ness, too. We won't give up until we've redefined dyslexia and every teacher is trained to spot, support and empower every dyslexic child.

Key Points

1. Dyslexics are often driven by a desire to make the world better, fairer.
2. We're not afraid to challenge the status quo.
3. Because we see things differently, we can solve problems innovatively.
4. We use our Dyslexic Strength of Communication to explain issues to the wider world and galvanise support to change things for the better.
5. We are resilient – we are masters in overcoming adversity.

I've always been grateful for being dyslexic. You can do things slightly differently. I really believe that recognising people's Dyslexic Strengths can lead to doing better business, as well as helping individuals.

Nick Jones

#MadeByDyslexia

5 REASONS WHY DYSLEXICS MAKE GREAT ENTREPRENEURS

From Sir Richard Branson to the founder of IKEA, Ingvar Kamprad, from Jo Malone to Steve Jobs, each one possessed a unique ability to see the world differently. To ask 'what if?' and 'why not?'. To turn their passion into a successful business that redefined their sector.

And these entrepreneurs don't just jolt our society forward. They fuel our economy, too.

THE VALUE OF DYSLEXIA

In the United States, entrepreneurship plays a crucial role in the national economy, as well as creating jobs and fuelling growth. According to Ewing Marion Kauffman Foundation's 2017 'Growth Entrepreneurship' index,[2] new companies in the US create about 3 million new jobs per year, while in the UK, female entrepreneurs could contribute £180 billion to the economy alone.[3]

BBC research found that 60 per cent of self-made millionaires are dyslexic.[4] That's certainly true on the BBC's flagship show for entrepreneurs, *Dragons' Den*. In a previous series, 40 per cent of the panel were Made By Dyslexia: Peter Jones and Theo Paphitis. While on the show's US counterpart, *Shark Tank*, more than 50 per cent of the panel were Made By Dyslexia: Kevin O'Leary, Daymond John and Barbara Corcoran.

> ***Watch*** *FUBU brand creator, Daymond John, talk to LinkedIn's Daniel Roth, where he explains how his dyslexic, visual mind helps him to map business plans in his head:*

MAKING A DIFFERENCE

Being an entrepreneur is not just about building a successful business and having financial success. Social entrepreneurs do amazing things to make the world a better place too. It's this Dyslexic Thinking and entrepreneurial skill set that is helping me and my team to build Made By Dyslexia.

So why do dyslexics make such good entrepreneurs?

Here are five good reasons why dyslexics make great entrepreneurs:

1. Dyslexics think differently – the Dyslexic Thinking skill of Imagining

Dyslexic brains process information differently. We are naturally creative, good at problem-solving and talented communicators. Our heightened abilities in areas like Visualisation and Reasoning skills alongside our natural entrepreneurial traits, bring a fresh and intuitive perspective. Put simply, we see the world differently. We use these skills to dream big, imagine new solutions and innovate in ways that others couldn't conceive possible.

Sir Richard Branson says:

> ***My dyslexia has shaped Virgin right from the very beginning and imagination has been the key to many of our successes. It helped me think big but keep our messages simple. The business world often gets caught up in facts and figures – and while the details and data are important, the ability to dream, conceptualise and innovate is what sets the successful and the unsuccessful apart.***

Dyslexic minds may be restricted by our school system, wherein standardised testing create standardised thinking. But in the world of business, where thinking differently gives you a competitive edge, we focus on our strengths and flourish.

That's because creative thinking comes naturally to dyslexics. It helps us to approach old problems in new ways. Being unconventional in a same-same market helps us to disrupt industries and give customers an alternative.

Jo Malone, says:

> ***My dyslexia is not a disability, but an ability to think differently, and if this world needs anything at this moment, it is people who think differently. We've learnt how to see around walls and spot the potential in something that others don't.***

2. Dyslexics keep it simple – the Dyslexic Thinking skill of Reasoning

There's plenty of complexity in building your own business. However, dyslexics are brilliant at using their enhanced Reasoning skills to see the bigger picture and simplify things. This in turn can help them to be bold and act fast, capitalising on opportunity.

Nick Jones, founder of Soho House says:

> ***One great advantage of being dyslexic is simplification. Simplifying things allows for***

better decision-making and is a real help when running a company.

Watch *Nick Jones talk about how determination, imagination and simplification have helped him build Soho House, arguably the most successful, but definitely the coolest chain of private members clubs in the world:*

3. Dyslexics are great explainers and storytellers – the Dyslexic Thinking skill of Communicating

While it may be hard to cope with mountains of paperwork, we are adept at creating clear messages that win hearts and minds. Dyslexics have an enhanced ability to simplify the narrative and sell the vision.

IKEA founder Ingvar Kamprad used his Dyslexic Thinking to create some interesting innovations. Take the unique names of IKEA's furniture for example. Having started IKEA as a mail-order sales business, his products were identified by individual codes. As many dyslexics would, he struggled to remember the numbers. So he decided to create a new system, naming each set of furniture after memorable Swedish names and places. The system has been used ever since and is renowned around the world.

Then consider the distinct assembly instructions for IKEA products. They are all pictures, no words. For a dyslexic who sees the world in a visual way, that makes perfect sense. It also became an iconic part of IKEA's appeal.

4. Dyslexics are passionate and curious – the Dyslexic Thinking skill of Exploring

Dyslexics are curious and questioning, building businesses that are fuelled by our passion and curiosity. We explore ideas in an energetic and constant way. And, when it comes to customer experience, we are often motivated to go the extra mile. As Nick Jones, Founder and CEO Soho House explains:

> ***To be successful in business you need to get your P's in the right order and dyslexia helps you do that. First 'passion', second great 'people', third great 'product'. Then 'profit' will follow.***

Dyslexics have a unique ability to explore and visualise outcomes, which can include multiple possibilities or multiple perspectives in business. They can imagine how a certain scenario will pan out, spot gaps and opportunities that others may miss. Or visualise a product from all angles. This gives them an amazing advantage when it comes to designing new products, inventing new services or improving existing products on the market.

5. Dyslexics are 'people' people – the Dyslexic Thinking skill of Connecting

Another skill that sets dyslexic entrepreneurs apart is their ability to motivate, lead and inspire people. This is born out of our strong Connecting skills and heightened emotional intelligence.

Being aware of our weaknesses and the need to focus on our strengths, we also become expert delegators. Sara Blakely, Founder and CEO of Spanx, who is also Made By Dyslexia, says:

The smartest thing I ever did was to hire my weakness.

By having this greater understanding of ourselves and others, we're able to create brilliant teams to grow companies faster.

And when it comes to communicating with our customers, our high levels of emotional intelligence, empathy and passion mean we are great at understanding how to reach and inspire them. This builds brands and products that truly connect with customers in a powerful authentic way.

One amazing example of this is Jamie Oliver, whose passion and enthusiasm shines through in his books and TV shows, motivates millions around the world – young and old – to cook.

> ***Watch*** *Jamie Oliver's Made By Dyslexia interview here:*

NEXT GENERATION ENTREPRENEURS MADE BY DYSLEXIA

So what does the future hold for dyslexic entrepreneurs? Well, with the right support and the right opportunities, dyslexic entrepreneurs will continue to transform the world we live in.

It's vital we support everyone with dyslexia to realise their potential, starting at school and running right through to the world of work. We must celebrate their imagination, creativity and problem-solving – the skills our entrepreneurs need for the future.

Key Points

1. Dyslexics are industry game-changers and imaginative innovators.
2. We are adept at simplifying industries and offering consumers an alternative.
3. Dyslexics are master communicators who can sell their vision, simply and clearly.
4. Businesses Made By Dyslexia are fuelled by passion and curiosity.
5. Dyslexics are 'people' people – who know how to motivate, lead and inspire their teams, often delegating effectively.

We need the creatives, we need imagination, we need people telling stories.

Dr Maggie Aderin-Pocock

#MadeByDyslexia

5 REASONS WHY DYSLEXICS MAKE SKILLED COMMUNICATORS

Here's a fact: nine out of ten dyslexics have poor spelling, punctuation and grammar, but many are amazing communicators.[5]

From Pulitzer Prize-winning journalists to respected CNN news anchors, high-profile bishops to gifted space communicators, dyslexics use their curiosity and passion to explore the world, understand complex situations or facts and explain them to others in a way that's simple and easy to understand.

So why do dyslexics make such good communicators?

Here are five reasons why dyslexics make skilled communicators:

1. **Dyslexics make sense of the bigger picture – the Dyslexic Thinking skill of Reasoning**

The dyslexic brain is wired differently, so we are able to connect stories and see patterns in narratives where others may not. This makes us adept at understanding big ideas or evolving situations and explaining them to others.

Many of us become skilled journalists and TV presenters, helping our audience to make sense of world events and situations that are constantly changing. CNN news anchors Anderson Cooper and Robyn Curnow are both Made By Dyslexia.

Thinking about his role as a storyteller, CNN news anchor Anderson Cooper says:

A lot of compelling stories in the world aren't being told, and the fact that people don't know about them compounds the suffering.

Robyn Curnow, says:

Generally, TV news is an amazing place to trust your dyslexic instincts. You have to look at the big picture, identify the story, tell the story and create a narrative that's simplified, so that an audience can understand the main issues.

Like four out of five people, Robyn Curnow attributes her success to her Dyslexic Strengths:

To write for television news is like a dyslexic dream . . . the sentences are simple, you're writing to pictures and you need to take away all the useless information. It has to be the real essence of the story.

Her ability to quickly summarise a situation, or assess the facts and present an angle, comes as a result of her dyslexic communication skills.

> ***Watch*** *Robyn Curnow explain why her greatest weakness is also her greatest strength in this interview with Made By Dyslexia:*

2. Dyslexics are great at simplifying – the Dyslexic Thinking skills of Reasoning and Communicating

Dyslexic minds are great at stripping away unnecessary detail to create clear, compelling messages. This means they excel in careers where explaining, educating or influencing are key, like teaching, marketing, journalism, campaigning or PR.

Roland Rudd, Founder and Chairman of PR firm Finsbury explains:

Being dyslexic enables you to simplify things very quickly. It enabled me to see the big picture and I could make decisions more creatively and effectively as a result.

Other dyslexic minds, like that of space scientist and communicator Dr Maggie Aderin-Pocock, use their dyslexic communication skills to simplify concepts that are 'out of this world' and go on to engage new audiences and inspire a generation. She explains:

As a scientist, I have found that I am able to take complex ideas and simplify them, story-tell and bring science ideas to life in my own unique way, this has been a huge advantage.

3. Dyslexics have high levels of empathy – the Dyslexic Thinking skill of Connecting

It isn't just our knack of making complex ideas clearer that makes us strong communicators. We're also able to use our high levels of empathy and emotional intelligence to create messages that are compelling too.

Gareth Cook, a journalist who is Made By Dyslexia and writes for the *New York Times Magazine* and *Boston Globe*, won the Pulitzer Prize in 2005 for 'explaining, with clarity and humanity, the complex scientific and ethical dimensions of stem-cell research.'

Dyslexics have a greater ability to sense, understand and respond to how others feel. This allows for a more authentic connection with people and can result in a deeper understanding of their stories and a greater skill in telling them. It's all part of our Connecting skills.

The Rt Revd, Sarah Mullally, Bishop of London, recognises the strengths her dyslexia brings:

> ***I love listening and solving problems. I also have a high level of emotional intelligence. I will respond differently to situations than other people.***

Watch *the 'People' People D.Spot vodcast with Bishop Sarah and Ruth May, Chief Nursing Officer for England and hear how their Dyslexic Thinking helped them guide two iconic institutions through a global pandemic:*

Empathy and emotional intelligence featured highly in Bishop Sarah's previous life, too. Before her ordination, she was England's Chief Nursing Officer. With these enhanced emotional strengths, it's no surprise that many dyslexics are drawn to careers like nursing, caring, social work and becoming champions of the socially disadvantaged. In fact, Dame Martina Milburn, Group Chief Executive of The Prince's Trust and former Chair of the Social Mobility Commission, is also Made By Dyslexia.

4. Dyslexics are passionate and curious – the Dyslexic Thinking skill of Exploring

What really makes dyslexics amazing communicators is our passion and curiosity. We love learning new things. And the energy and passion we use to do it inspires others.

Jamie Oliver's infectious energy and skill in communicating has made even the most complex recipes simple and easy for most of us to have a go at in our own kitchens. In this way, he's able to pass on his passion and curiosity to millions of us around the world.

My strength is a complete obsession and expression to empower and teach people to cook. Whether it's a book, the paper it's on, the photographer we use – the aim is to

create something that empowers everyone to create food that's affordable, which a king would eat.

5. Dyslexics engage hearts and minds – the Dyslexic Thinking skill of Connecting

The combination of being able to make sense of the bigger picture, simplify complex ideas, use our emotional intelligence and inspire people with our passion and curiosity means we are great at engaging hearts and minds. We know how to entertain, inspire, motivate and influence people.

Dav Pilkey, the creator of *Captain Underpants*, says his dyslexia and other learning abilities:

Helped me to write stories that were not boring. It helped me to choose my words very, very carefully.

His words (and pictures) have helped millions of children (dyslexic or not) love reading.

Communication skills are crucial to the future economy and world of work that humans will find themselves in.

Technology and machines are already taking over the elements dyslexics have found challenging, like spelling, punctuation and grammar (rarely signs of creativity in themselves), so we can focus on our

Dyslexic Strengths of crafting clear, compelling messages that inspire, motivate, educate and drive change around the world.

Key Points

1. Dyslexics see the big picture. They are good at understanding evolving situations and explaining them to others.
2. Dyslexics are great at simplifying – that makes them good at explaining, educating or influencing.
3. We use our high levels of empathy and emotional intelligence to connect with others.
4. Our passion for things is infectious, and we inspire others to love those things too.
5. Dyslexics are skilled at engaging hearts and minds.

The world is changing. And imagination is key to everything.

Keira Knightley

#MadeByDyslexia

5 REASONS WHY DYSLEXICS MAKE GREAT IMAGINERS

Dyslexic brains have changed the world with revolutionary art, music, architecture and ideas. From John Lennon to Pablo Picasso, Albert Einstein to Agatha Christie, Steven Spielberg to Steve McQueen, these people have used their imagination to kickstart movements, create characters and produce films that have taken us to lands we couldn't have otherwise imagined.

BUT WHAT MAKES DYSLEXICS THINK DIFFERENTLY?

Dyslexic brains are 'wired' differently. The left parietal temporal area of our brains uses different neural pathways. That helps people with dyslexia to think differently, creatively, laterally.

Each dyslexic will have a different pattern of Strengths and Challenges. But for many who are born with the ability to imagine in innovative and inventive ways, they'll go on to transform the world we live in.

Here are five reasons why dyslexics make great imaginers:

1. Dyslexics see the world differently – the Dyslexic Thinking skill of Imagining

Dyslexic minds have used their imaginations to flourish in visual fields like design, architecture, photography and film. In fact, a study that took place at one of the UK's top art colleges, Central Saint Martins, found that up to 75 per cent of the 360 foundation-year students assessed had dyslexia. Many were in the top 10 per cent in the country for intelligence. And a large percentage had above average visual spatial skills.[6]

Dyslexic painters like Pablo Picasso reimagined the portrait and invented a whole new movement in art, while Tracey Emin made her dyslexic spelling part of her art.

2. Dyslexics are multisensory – the Dyslexic Thinking skill of Visualising

Dyslexics often experience the world with heightened senses: seeing patterns that others won't see, picking up on sounds or smells that others haven't noticed.

Composer, filmmaker and Turner Prize winner Steve McQueen says his creativity is more heightened because of his dyslexia:

Image and sound were much more heightened because my oral reading wasn't as good.

Watch *Steve McQueen talk about the benefits of being Made By Dyslexia here:*

3. Dyslexics create original ideas, never imagined before – the Dyslexic Thinking skill of Imagining

Dyslexic minds are brilliant at thinking in original, new ways. Dyslexic architect Richard Rogers turned the architecture world on its head when he built the Pompidou Centre in Paris – inside out. All the plumbing, electrics, air circulation, wires and pipes – and even the escalators – were on the outside of the building.

Watch *Richard Rogers, the world-famous architect, talk about being Made By Dyslexia here:*

Another of the world's most iconic and original buildings, the Sydney Opera House, was Made By Dyslexia, too. Dutch architect Jørn Utzon was inspired by sailing in Sydney Harbour, watching the crests of the waves and seeing the arc of the seagulls' wings.

4. Dyslexics are skilled storytellers – the Dyslexic Thinking skill of Communicating

Of course, dyslexics aren't just capable of reshaping the world around them. They're brilliant at imagining new ones, too. Skilled storytellers, they create vivid worlds, spin gripping stories and summon up unforgettable characters we love and empathise with.

Some, like Agatha Christie, create bestselling novels (her books have sold over a billion copies worldwide). Others, like poets W.B. Yeats and Benjamin Zephaniah, use language in new and surprising ways to help us see ordinary things in an extraordinary way.

5. Dyslexics imagine new worlds in film – the Dyslexic Thinking skill of Imagining

Using the power of their imaginations, it's no wonder that the film industry is full of talent that's Made By Dyslexia. From actors to film directors, they are experts at spinning stories, imagining worlds and creating films that engage all of our senses.

Steven Spielberg only realised he was Made By Dyslexia in his sixties. Speaking about it for the first time in 2012, he explained:

I'm in a business right now where reading is very important. It's of critical importance to me that I read books and scripts. And so, I've been able to overcompensate . . . it takes me 2 hours and 45 minutes to read what most people can read in 1 hour and 10 minutes. But I have great comprehension in what I do read, because I do read slowly. So I'm able to appreciate good writing.

Watch *Oscar-winning director Steven Spielberg talking about how he is Made By Dyslexia here:*

It's easy to lose ourselves in a world brought to life by talented actors and actresses, many of whom are also Made By Dyslexia. From Keira Knightley to Orlando Bloom, Sir Anthony Hopkins to Whoopi Goldberg, Jennifer Aniston to Will Smith, their Dyslexic Thinking skills allow them to fully imagine and realise the character they play.

Very often, finding and focusing on those strengths is a life-changing move for any dyslexic. Oscar-nominated actress Keira Knightley explains how acting 'was the carrot' that helped her through school.

***Watch** Keira Knightley's interview with Made By Dyslexia here:*

THE BEST IMAGINERS ON THE PLANET

Of course, when it comes to imagining, no one comes close to the imaginative power of children. Dyslexic children are born storytellers, elaborate explainers, wide-eyed make-believers and gifted entertainers. They use their imaginations in natural, unselfconscious ways.

But our school system is not designed to support this style of lateral, creative thinking. Instead they are forced down a route of linear learning, that focuses on linguistic ability (spelling, punctuation, written tests and exams). And yet, as the world of work changes, these creative, Imagining skills are more valued than ever.

The world needs Dyslexic Thinking. So that's why we're making it our mission to train every teacher to spot, support and empower the next generation of dyslexic Imaginers.

Key Points

1. Dyslexics have above average visual spatial skills – they quite literally see the world differently.
2. We experience the world with heightened senses – noticing details, sounds or smells that others miss.
3. Dyslexic minds are brilliant at thinking in original, new ways.
4. We are skilled storytellers, creating vivid worlds and unforgettable characters.
5. We thrive in the world of film, where we use all of our senses to engage others.

The moment you give up, is the moment you let someone else win.

Kobe Bryant

#MadeByDyslexia

5 REASONS WHY DYSLEXICS MAKE UNSTOPPABLE SPORTS CHAMPIONS

What gives a World Champion their edge? Talent? Skills? Perseverance? A will to win? How about being dyslexic?

Sports heavyweights like Muhammad Ali (three times World Boxing Champion), Sir Jackie Stewart (three times winner of the World Drivers' Championship) and basketball legend Magic Johnson (played for LA Lakers for 13 seasons) all had one thing in common: each one is Made By Dyslexia.

Here are five reasons why dyslexics make unstoppable sports champions:

1. **Strong visual memory – the Dyslexic Thinking skill of Visualising**

While dyslexics struggle to memorise facts, like times tables, spelling, punctuation or grammar rules, they have an incredibly strong visual memory – which can give them an unfair advantage on the sports field.

F1 racing World Champion, Sir Jackie Stewart, can visualise each twist and turn on every race track, saying:

The old Nürburgring had 187 corners per lap, and I can still give you every gear change, every braking distance on each of the 187 corners. But I can't say the alphabet.

He also puts his success down to picking up on small details that others might easily overlook and being able to communicate with his mechanics more clearly, which builds a stronger team.

Watch *our interview with Sir Jackie Stewart here:*

If you're dyslexic, understanding how your brain thinks is the key to harnessing your potential, both on and off the sports pitch.

Former England rugby captain, Chris Robshaw, explains he needs to see a play on the pitch, rather than study it in the team room, to understand it better:

I'm a very visual person. I need to go through bits, whereas other people like to read, they like to listen to stuff. I could sit in a meeting room and we could talk about our plays and our line outs, whatever it be . . . and a lot of that won't go in. However, if I go out on a pitch and run through it once, it will all go in and I'll be completely fine.

Similarly, Tim Tebow, champion NFL quarterback, taught himself game plays by using flash cards before big games – while the rest of the team would memorise complicated playbooks.

2. Perseverance – the Dyslexic Thinking skill of Exploring

Four in five dyslexics said that knowing they were dyslexic helped them develop the perseverance needed to succeed.[7] Take Olympic Gold medal winner Caitlin Jenner.

She said:

If I wasn't dyslexic, I probably wouldn't have won the Games. If I had been a better reader, then that would have come easily, sports

would have come easily, and I never would have realised that the way you get ahead in life is hard work.

Current Olympic shot-put champion Michelle Carter agrees. Talking to Understood, she says:

You can do whatever you set your mind to – you just may do it differently. You may have to work a little bit harder, but you can do it.

And while many people might think skill gives champions their edge, the world's greatest boxer, Muhammad Ali, believes otherwise:

Champions aren't made in gyms. Champions are made from something they have deep inside them – a desire, a dream, a vision. They have to have the skill, and the will. But the will must be stronger than the skill.

Dyslexics are masters at working harder in order to succeed, developing grit, determination and resilience along the way. And, as our 'Value of Dyslexia' reports from 2018[8] and 2019[9] show, these skills, along with problem-solving, creative thinking, communication and leadership, are the skills that are vital to the future workplace, not just the sports field.

Watch *a summary of our* 'Value of Dyslexia' *reports and see how Dyslexic Thinking skills are exactly the skills needed for the future world of work:*

3. Intuition – the Dyslexic Thinking skill of Visualising

Many dyslexics have strong visualisation skills. And when it comes to sport, this can translate to an uncanny knack of knowing how the game is going to unfold, or where the play is going to take place, which often influences the result of the game.

Children at Millfield School, which specialises in sport and dyslexia, say:

It's like a superpower in a way, because you can see things that other people can't.

They explain:

I'm better at hockey, because I know where to stand in the pitch because I understand the game better.

***Watch** the full* 'Dyslexia Awareness: Dyslexic Strengths' *film here:*

Josh Clark, Head of The Schenck School, Atlanta, Georgia (which specialises in dyslexic teaching) describes dyslexic children's intuitive ability like this:

> ***They could be the child on the sports field, that seems to have this premonition of how things are going to work. The child that can predict where the ball is going to go. Or know when to move left when everyone else moves right, because they understand that's how the play is going to come about.***

This kind of intuitive skill leads to an ability to be in the right place at the right time, which can change the course of a game, whether that's top-flight rugby, Premier League football, NFL or more.

4. Exceptional focus – the Dyslexic Thinking skill of Exploring

While it's true that some dyslexics find it easy to get distracted and need support to stay on task, many can become fully absorbed in a passion.

When it comes to elite athletes, this ability to focus and stay calm when the stakes are high and the pressure is on, is crucial to their success.

Mo Farah is the most successful British track athlete in modern Olympic Games history, winning the Olympic Gold medal in both the 5,000m and 10,000m in 2012 and 2016. Mo Farah explains:

If I don't train, I don't win. If I don't focus, I don't win.

Vancouver-based neurotherapist Mari Swingle, author of *i-Minds: How Cell Phones, Computers, Gaming and Social Media Are Changing Our Brains, Our Behaviour and the Evolution of Our Species*, says a dyslexic mind can display exceptional focus when they 'get in the zone', which leads to extraordinary calmness that allows them to outperform others.[10]

Rashan Gary, NFL star and outside linebacker with the Green Bay Packers, says:

Having dyslexia means I go above and beyond in whatever I put my mind to. Failure has never been an option for me.

5. Spatial awareness – the Dyslexic Thinking skill of Visualising

Finally, thanks to their visualisation skills, dyslexic sports stars develop an extraordinary perception of the space around them. This includes their relationship to others on the pitch, track or stage and helps them to make decisions about how and where to move next.

Mari Swingle says:

> ***There's a different form of spatial perception that dyslexics have, so it's almost fundamentally what hurts them in their learning to read actually helps them on courses and tracks.***

This ability to visualise, or see how set pieces should play out, is particularly useful to former England rugby captain, Chris Robshaw:

> ***Wherever I'm playing, for club or country, I'll sit down the night before and just take 15 minutes going through the plays and I'll actually picture myself where I need to be at this play, where I'm going next, so you actually see it all, and for me that's my best way of learning.***

These powerful visualisation skills help dyslexics approach the game differently, and give them an added advantage over others on the pitch.

Key Points

1. Dyslexics have a strong visual memory. They think in pictures rather than words.
2. Dyslexics have high levels of perseverance, grit and determination.
3. On the sports pitch, our intuition gives us a sense of where the ball will go next or how the game is going to unfold.
4. A dyslexic mind can display exceptional focus, which helps them outperform others.
5. Thanks to their visualisation skills, dyslexic sports stars develop an extraordinary perception of the space around them.

Dyslexia is the single biggest driver of ingenuity, imagination and scientific achievement in history.

The Rt Hon Matt Hancock MP

#MadeByDyslexia

DYSLEXIC INVENTIONS – 5 OF THE GREATEST BREAKTHROUGHS MADE BY DYSLEXIA

Imagine a world without Dyslexic Thinking. There'd be no phones, no cars, no aeroplanes, no light bulb.

Here are five items we couldn't live without – each one Made By Dyslexia:

1. THE IPHONE

Created by Apple CEO, Steve Jobs and Apple Chief of Design, Jony Ive – both Made By Dyslexia.

- The iPhone revolutionised mobile phones and changed the way we communicate in the twenty-first century.
- The simple, iconic design ensured we could make calls, check emails, access the Internet, photograph the world and take our entire music collection with us in our pocket, anywhere we go.
- Steve Jobs was a visionary imaginer, a master of simplifying the big idea and an inspirational

speaker and leader – all key Dyslexic Thinking skills.

- Fellow dyslexic and creator Jony Ive has dedicated his career to simplifying design to the beauty of its essentials, creating iconic products that are simple and joyful to use.

2. THE AEROPLANE

Created by the Wright brothers, both Made By Dyslexia.

- Orville and Wilbur Wright used their Dyslexic Thinking skills of Imagining, Visualising and Exploring to create the first powered, manned, flying machine in 1903.
- Though they had many setbacks along the way, their grit and determination meant they became the first people to invent, build and fly the world's first successful motor-operated plane.
- What made their planes so successful was the three-axis control, which is still used in aeroplanes today.

Every once in a while, a revolutionary product comes along that changes everything. Today Apple is going to reinvent the phone and here it is.

Steve Jobs

#MadeByDyslexia

3. THE CAR

Created by Henry Ford, Made By Dyslexia.

- Henry Ford was a dyslexic game-changer who produced the first Ford Model T car in 1908 and revolutionised the motor industry.
- He was the first person to make automobiles affordable to the many, by inventing the assembly line technique of mass production.
- These mass production techniques are now used across the world to produce almost everything we buy.
- His Dyslexic Thinking skills of Visualising, Reasoning and Imagining allowed him to creatively problem-solve and innovate in ways that continue to transform the world we live in today.

4. THE LIGHT BULB

Created by Thomas Edison, Made By Dyslexia.

- Thomas Edison is described as America's most prolific inventor, with over 1,093 US patents to his name.
- His Dyslexic Thinking skills of Exploring, Reasoning and Imagining helped him to discover everything from the light bulb to the phonograph (gramophone or record player).
- He also invented an early form of video camera (called a motion picture camera) and a type of rechargeable battery.

If we all worked on the assumption that what is accepted as true is really true, there would be little hope of advance.

Orville Wright

#MadeByDyslexia

5. THE TELEPHONE

Created by Alexander Graham Bell, Made By Dyslexia.

- Today, it's easy to take for granted our ability to pick up the phone and talk.
- But it was Alexander Graham Bell's dyslexic skills of Visualising, Exploring and Reasoning that allowed him to connect the dots and invent a way to transmit sound over a network of telegraph wires.
- His discovery transformed our ability to communicate, regardless of space and time, changing life for centuries after.

Key Points

1. Dyslexia is the single biggest driver of innovation, from the iPhone to the aeroplane.
2. Dyslexics are highly original thinkers who ask 'what if?' and 'why not?'.
3. Dyslexics have a natural ability to simplify, creating revolutionary products we can't live without.
4. Dyslexics are not afraid to fail.
5. Their determination feeds their passion for innovation.

There is no man living that cannot do more than he thinks he can.

Henry Ford

#MadeByDyslexia

I have not failed. I've just found 10,000 ways that won't work.

Thomas Edison

#MadeByDyslexia

The day is coming when telegraph wires will be laid onto houses just like water or gas – and friends converse with each other without leaving home.

Alexander Graham Bell

#MadeByDyslexia

What we shouldn't do is employ Superwoman and spend our time telling her how bad she is with Kryptonite.

Steve Varley

#MadeByDyslexia

DYSLEXIA IN THE WORKPLACE – 5 TOP TIPS FROM OUR COMMUNITY

We asked the Made By Dyslexia community around the world to share a range of top tips for success in the workplace.

Firstly, let's refresh our memory and look at the Dyslexic Strengths and Challenges that dyslexics face in the workplace:

5 WAYS DYSLEXIC THINKING HELPS YOU IN YOUR JOB

1. Make connections across complex issues, subjects and data, which others don't see.
2. Cut through the noise and see the big picture, rather than getting stuck in the detail.
3. Communicate and explain complex subjects through storytelling and simplifying.
4. Solve problems in different ways, coming up with new ideas to tackle them.
5. Build, support and empower teams, people and organisations.

5 THINGS DYSLEXICS STRUGGLE WITH IN THE WORKPLACE

1. Information overload, especially via email.
2. Competing or unclear priorities.
3. Long and complicated meetings, being asked to write on a flip chart or read aloud.
4. Too much information in written form – not enough visual presentation of information.
5. Tiredness or anxiety due to the effort of working at high pace.

Now, let's see what the Made By Dyslexia community suggested:

5 WAYS TO OVERCOME THOSE STRUGGLES

1. Be upfront with colleagues and managers. Explain your Dyslexic Strengths and Challenges.
2. Use assistive technology, like speech-to-text programmes.
3. Ask for reasonable adjustments in workplace assessments (for example, extra time).
4. Find methods of organisation that work for you.
5. Have a supportive team around you with different strengths.

5 WAYS TECHNOLOGY HELPS

1. Text-to-speech allows you to proofread documents and read long text without fatigue.
2. Tablets allow you to take notes and store them easily.
3. Automated meeting requests make arrangements easier, without the high mental load of remembering times, places, people and topics.
4. Automated search and filing helps you find things without having to use a complicated filing system.
5. Using dictation software to create documents, like Dictate or Immersive Reader in Office 365.

5 THINGS EVERY MANAGER SHOULD KNOW ABOUT DYSLEXIA

1. The benefits, including big-picture thinking, seeing things from another point of view and spotting patterns are dyslexic skills and are the skills of the future.
2. Most workplaces show unconscious bias towards dyslexic people.

3. Dyslexics can be a huge asset if you work out how to get the best from them.
4. Simple adjustments can help dyslexics to fly.
5. Dyslexics have the skills needed by most organisations of the future.

5 THINGS EVERY MANAGER CAN DO TO HELP

1. Understand what dyslexia means for that person, their pattern of Strengths and Challenges.
2. Dyslexics need encouragement and support, not sanction, if things are not going well; often they will already have anxiety about performance.
3. Avoid trigger words like 'lazy, sloppy, careless, scatty' – dyslexics are none of these things. If they appear like that, it's a sign they need more help.
4. Give dyslexics the big picture and watch them make it a reality.
5. Use bullets and summaries to share key information.

5 TOP TIPS FOR ANY DYSLEXIC EMPLOYEE

1. Work out what dyslexia means for you – your Strengths and your Challenges.
2. Be upfront with others and don't be embarrassed or wait until you hit a problem.
3. You will be very good at your Dyslexic Strengths, which will benefit your employer.
4. Ask for what you need. Don't just overwork to get through; you will burn out.
5. If systems don't work for you, constructively see if they can be changed.

5 TOP TIPS FOR EVERY EMPLOYER

1. Dyslexics are an asset to the organisation – treasure them.
2. Your workplace probably prevents them from doing their best work, try to change it.
3. Listen and respond to what they need, even if it seems strange.
4. Summarise large documents into bullets and summaries.

5. Present information in a multisensory way, using videos, pictures and diagrams rather than too much text.

5 TOP THINGS THAT WOULD HELP DURING THE JOB APPLICATION/ RECRUITMENT PROCESS

1. Offer the basics – extra time, quiet rooms for examinations, clear questions.
2. Forgive typos and spelling – they are not a reflection of commitment or ability.
3. Understand that tests and interviews don't always showcase a dyslexic's full skills and talents. Help them to show their abilities in different ways.
4. Encourage applicants to tell you they're dyslexic by acknowledging that you value Dyslexic Thinking.
5. Don't insist on a formal assessment to trigger reasonable adjustments, a self-declaration of dyslexia should be enough.

The most important thing is to try and inspire people so that they can be great in whatever they want to do.

Kobe Bryant

#MadeByDyslexia

In every classroom, in every school, across the world, there are one in five kids with exactly the thinking the future needs.

Kate Griggs

#MadeByDyslexia

PART 4:

THIS is Dyslexia in Kids

Find out what dyslexic kids are interested in, what they love, what they're passionate about. And . . . let them loose! And they can be absolutely exceptional in the areas of their passions.

Sir Richard Branson

#MadeByDyslexia

HOW TO SPOT, SUPPORT AND EMPOWER DYSLEXIC CHILDREN

What's it like to be a child who is Made By Dyslexia? Well, like adults, dyslexic kids have their own unique pattern of Strengths and Challenges and the key to success for our dyslexic children is to spot and support these early.

But *the* most important thing we can do for our dyslexic children is to find out what they are extraordinarily good at and are passionate about, and help them to do lots of it, because therein lies the formula for unleashing their Dyslexic Superpowers.

HOW TO SPOT THE STRENGTHS

When I was nine years old, my life was transformed when a teacher saw past my test scores and recognised my Strengths, and what I was passionate about. These Strengths and passions are the very things that help me succeed in my role today, and I use them every day to do something that I absolutely love.

I have seen the same 'success formula' in thousands of dyslexic people, young and old. It's the formula I encouraged with my own children, which has led them into fulfilling careers too.

This is what drives me to help everyone spot and support Dyslexic Strengths today.

How to SPOT your child's Dyslexic Superpower

- Think about what your child loves to do and would do for hours, if left to their own devices. These are usually their Dyslexic Thinking skills.
- Find out what they are passionate about, what they love to talk about, watch or learn about.
- Encourage them to do both of the above, lots and lots. Skill + Practice + Passion = Superpower.
- Easy-to-spot strengths include sport, art, music, dancing. But empathy, kindness, imagining, listening and questioning are all incredibly valuable superpowers too.
- Acknowledge their expertise. Dyslexics often don't realise how good they are at these things, so may not recognise them as their Superpowers.

My Strength is just a complete obsession with any expression of empowering people and teaching people to cook, and it's that simple.

Jamie Oliver

#MadeByDyslexia

SPOTTING EXPERTISE

Dyslexic kids become experts in the subjects they love because they are inquisitive and curious and use lots of Dyslexic Thinking skills, like Exploring and Questioning, to find out all there is to know about it. This is often a great way to spot dyslexia in our kids early. Just observe how they master a topic they love, but at the same time struggle to grasp simple skills their peers find easy. This mismatch or 'spiky profile' is a key marker for dyslexia and can often be spotted at a very young age.

For example, my son Ted was a dinosaur 'expert' when he was aged four. He devoured dinosaur magazines, TV shows and films. He knew the name of every single dinosaur, whether they were herbivore or carnivore and would draw amazing pictures of them too. But he just wasn't interested in or couldn't grasp reading or writing at all. This was the point I knew for sure he was dyslexic.

Finding and focusing on our strengths is key to our success. It helps us build self-esteem and often uncovers lifelong passions that we turn into successful, rewarding careers – if we are encouraged and supported along the way.

An amazing example of this is the palaeontologist Jack Horner. Jack flunked his exams over and over but continued to apply to every palaeontology department in the US. However, without qualifications, none would hire him. This didn't deter him; instead he spent his time exploring and discovering, building an extensive collection of dinosaur bones and dinosaur eggs until he could eventually crack open enough eggs to find an embryo! Jack become the first person ever to discover the dinosaur embryo. Now everyone wanted to hire him, and Jack went on to become an award-winning scientist, one of the world leaders in his field, and even became the dinosaur advisor on the *Jurassic Park* movies.

Watch *the wonderful interview with Jack Horner filmed at a dinosaur dig in Montana here:*

BUILDING SELF-ESTEEM

Spotting Dyslexic Thinking and focusing on our Strengths is key to building self-esteem. Because otherwise, we lose confidence in ourselves and our ability to learn. There is a real danger that when children find things challenging that their friends find easy, they lose heart and mistakenly believe they are less able or less intelligent than their peers (when neither is the case).

With education's emphasis on measuring things that dyslexics find challenging, like reading, writing, spelling and rote learning, it is no surprise that dyslexic children grow up acutely aware of the things they CAN'T do, instead of treasuring the things they CAN do.

This feeling can be created right from the start of their education. Research found:

- One in three dyslexic children aged 5–6 years already feel they can't keep up or do the things other children can.[1]
- By ages 7–8 that figure increases to two in three.[2]

SUPPORTING WITH POSITIVE PRAISE

Research suggests that we are most motivated to improve when we hear negative and positive comments in a ratio of 1:5. That's five pieces of praise for every one negative comment. It's true in teaching, as research from Sabey, Charlton and Charlton highlights.[3] And it's true in relationships and workplaces as Jack Zenger and Joseph

Folkman point out in their article 'The Ideal Praise-to-Criticism Ratio'.[4]

Positive praise is vital for dyslexic children. And even if certain things are challenging, or progress is slow, each small win should be celebrated. It's vital to acknowledge and highlight Dyslexic Strengths in every dyslexic child, so these children can experience the success they deserve too.

EMPOWERING DYSLEXIC THINKERS

Not only is finding and focusing on our strengths crucial to building positive self-esteem but it will help us find the careers that we'll be successful at and feel fulfilled in.

Twelve-year-old vegan chef, CBBC presenter and YouTube star Omari McQueen found that school and his extraordinary dyslexic mind didn't quite fit. But then he discovered his passion for cooking at home. Now, he runs his own vegan dip company, presents a CBBC TV cookery show, hosts his own YouTube channel and is in the process of writing a cookbook. Proving, of course, that when dyslexic children are empowered to find and focus on their Strengths, they are truly unstoppable.

Watch *our brilliant interview with Omari McQueen here:*

Attitude is a little thing that makes a big difference.

Winston Churchill

#MadeByDyslexia

All children are artists, the problem is how to remain one when you grow up.

Pablo Picasso

#MadeByDyslexia

I wish teachers were more aware of the yin and yang with dyslexia. There are some challenges: the written word, spelling, things like that are more difficult for dyslexics. But the imagination, the storytelling, the communication, the empathy, all these positives are sometimes neglected within the school system.

Dr Maggie Aderin-Pocock

#MadeByDyslexia

CONNECT THE SPOTS

We need to spot and nurture the Dyslexic Strengths of children in every classroom, in every school, right around the world. After all, these children have the **exact** skills the future needs.

We've known how to spot, support and empower dyslexic learners since the 1930s. But despite there being one in five dyslexic children in every classroom, around the world, teachers are still not routinely trained in dyslexia.

Research suggests:

- 98 per cent of parents and teachers say teachers need more training in how to identify and support dyslexia.[5]
- 91 per cent of parents and teachers say their school needs a better understanding and recognition of Dyslexic Strengths.[6]
- 80 per cent of dyslexic children leave school without being spotted.[7]

That's why Made By Dyslexia has partnered with Microsoft to create FREE online dyslexia awareness training to enable every teacher to spot, support and empower EVERY dyslexic student. In 2020, we launched our Connect the Spots campaign with a mission to train EVERY teacher in the world by 2025.

The training is video-based and perfect for teachers and parents, packed full of useful tips from expert teachers. It's inspiring and empowering. We have links to some of the films in the relevant sections of the book, but you can watch them all via the links below.

WHAT HAPPENS WHEN WE FAIL TO SPOT THE STRENGTHS?

Failing to spot dyslexia results in low self-esteem in childhood and carries on into adult life. Not being taught to recognise their valuable way of thinking, and using it to their advantage, means many dyslexics never fully realise their potential. And that is something we can and MUST change.

Watch *our D.Spot vodcast* 'Dyslexic Superpowers' *with three amazing educators who are empowering their students' Dyslexic Strengths here:*

Useful links:

Learn more about the Connect the Spots campaign in this report.

***Watch** our* 'Connect the Spots: Training Teachers to Empower Dyslexic Children' *film here:*

Learn more on the parents and teachers pages on our website at www.madebydyslexia.org

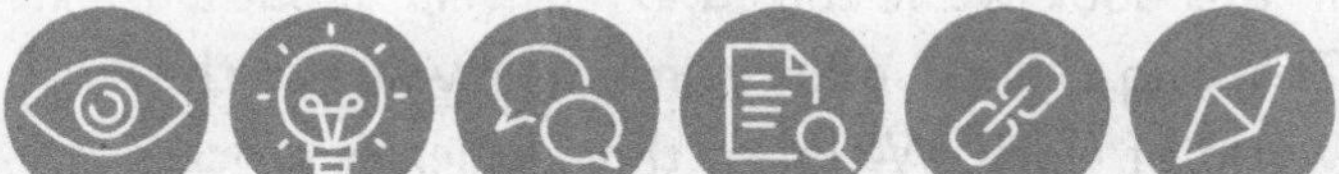

There are different types of intelligence and everyone has the ability to be brilliant.

Jamie Oliver

#MadeByDyslexia

DYSLEXIC THINKING SKILLS IN CHILDREN EXPLAINED

In this book we've talked extensively about Dyslexic Thinking skills in adults and their value to the world of work. We know that dyslexics process information differently, and that this difference results in a pattern of Strengths and Challenges, which are different for every person. This is exactly the same in dyslexic children.

To identify Dyslexic Thinking skills in children, we conducted one of the largest research projects of its kind. Our extensive research with dyslexic people, teachers, psychologists and parents, helped us to gather a unique insight into Dyslexic Strengths and thinking skills in children. These are the things that dyslexic children are naturally good at, and love to do. Because they love to do them so much, they practise them lots and become extraordinarily good at them and they become their Superpowers.

Skill + Practice + Passion = Superpower

From this research, we developed 7 Archetypes:

1. **Storytellers**
2. **Makers**
3. **Entertainers**
4. **Movers**
5. **Imaginers**
6. **Questioners**
7. **'People' People**

The 7 Archetypes are designed as children's characters who bring these Dyslexic Thinking skills to life by explaining them in a way that's relatable for children, their parents and their teachers.

***Watch** HRH Princess Beatrice read*
Xtraordinary People:

7 THINKING SKILLS ARCHETYPES

Dyslexic children have a natural ability in some or all of the following 7 Archetypes.

While all children will show ability and interest in these areas, dyslexics tend to immerse themselves and become very good, often 'expert' at them.

You can develop resilient confident learners by nurturing these natural abilities, which can develop into valuable skills in work and life.

Storytellers

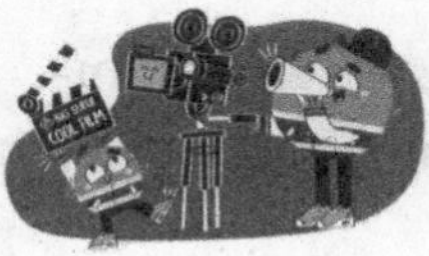

Makers

Entertainers

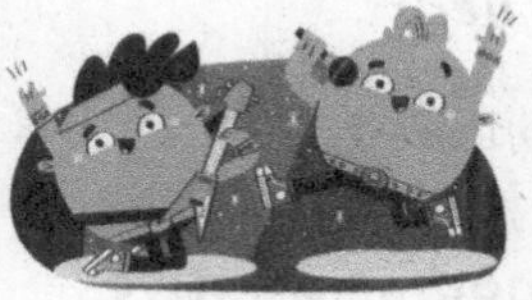

Movers

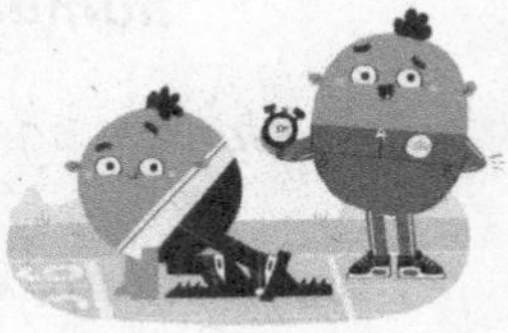

Imaginers

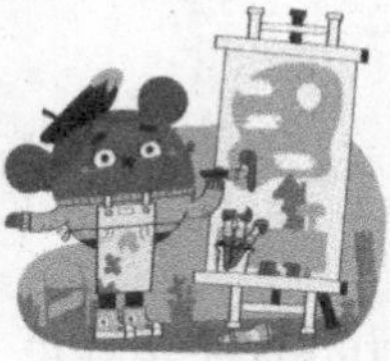

Questioners

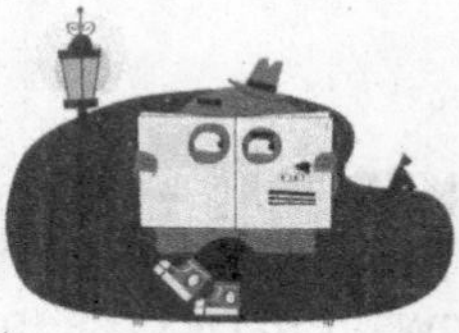

'People' People

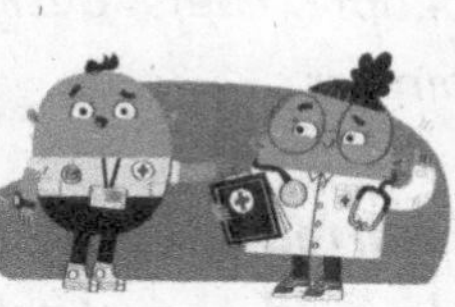

STORYTELLERS

Persuasive. Tell tall tales. Elaborate explainers. Invent stories. Love stories and films.

When they grow up, Storytellers often become journalists, teachers, writers, filmmakers, politicians or campaigners.

My Dyslexic Superpower is imagining while I'm writing . . . and I have a humungous heart.

Janice, age 8, Tennessee, US

I was always very good at creative writing, I was always top of those classes.

Keira Knightley

MAKERS

Jigsaws. Puzzles. Lego. Building things. Making things. Cooking. Crafts. Art and painting.

When they grow up, Makers often become architects, craftspeople, chefs, designers, gardeners, artists or programmers.

When I started cooking my mum vegan meals, and she started getting

much better, I got happier and it's like cooking was my escape.

Omari McQueen, age 12, London, UK

My Strength is just a complete obsession with any expression of empowering people and teaching people to cook, and it's that simple.

Jamie Oliver

ENTERTAINERS

Music and rhythm. Singing. Dancing. Jokers. Expressive arts. Like putting on a show.

When they grow up, Entertainers often become actors, musicians, comedians, salespeople, PR people or presenters.

I'm a rapper, so the way I express myself is through rapping.

Joe, age 14, London, UK

My mother sent me to dance class when I was five . . . as soon as I realised that I had a strength in it, then I excelled and that changed my whole attitude to everything else I approached.

Dame Darcey Bussell

MOVERS

Fidgets 'on the go'. Physical risk takers. Sports/ball skills. Balance. Climbing. Skateboarding. Gymnastics.

When they grow up, Movers often become musicians, sportspeople, dancers, sports coaches, choreographers or firefighters.

My Superpower is sport. When I'm struggling at school it helps me feel confident.

Archie, age 11, Worcester, UK

I found happiness and I found my confidence on the rugby pitch.

Chris Robshaw, former England rugby captain

IMAGINERS

Daydreaming. Making up games and fantasy/imaginary worlds. Create dens and 'worlds' out of things. Get lost in their imagination, immersed in activities.

When they grow up, Imaginers often become scientists, inventors, entrepreneurs, artists, actors, photographers or filmmakers.

One of my Dyslexic Superpowers is I love to do filmmaking. I love all the behind the scenes of it, I especially like doing the

make-up, the hair, the wardrobe. I love filming and I love creating new movies and ideas

Elsa, age 13, Chicago, US

I don't dream at night, I dream at day, I dream all day – I'm dreaming for a living.

Steven Spielberg

QUESTIONERS

Constantly ask 'what if?' and 'why not?, Challenge norms and rules. Have an answer for everything. Always curious. Problem-solvers. Explain things to everyone.

When they grow up, Questioners often become detectives, spies, entrepreneurs, journalists, writers or change-makers.

My Dyslexic Superpower is curiosity. I am curious and I ask a lot of questions. I ask until I know all the information I need to know.

Elena, age 14, Sicily, Italy

We are curious, we're creative, I think, we can simplify things . . . see the big picture . . . and I think in the end we 'connect the dots'.

Sir Richard Branson

'PEOPLE' PEOPLE

Peacemakers. Social organisers. Busybodies. Helpers. Charmers. Carers. Leaders.

When they grow up, 'People' People often become nurses, doctors, teachers, care workers, managers or presenters.

My Dyslexic Superpower is . . . when someone walks into a room, I can feel their emotion straight away and I know what they are feeling. I can just feel what they feel.

Hope, age 7, York, UK

For me, that empathy with people, has always been at the heart of who I am, which is something that's attributed to dyslexic thinking.

The Rt Revd, Sarah Mullally

Watch *dyslexic children around the world explain their Dyslexic Superpowers:*

XTRAORDINARY PEOPLE QUIZ

What type of Xtraordinary person are you? What do you love to do? What are you naturally good at? Tick the descriptions that sound like you to find out.

Storytellers

- ❍ You love to invent stories. Characters and adventures just pop out of your brain.
- ❍ You love to listen to stories and always ask for one more before bed.
- ❍ You're good at persuading people to do things.
- ❍ You're good at explaining things.

Makers

- ❍ You just love Lego and build all sorts of amazing creations.
- ❍ You're brilliant at jigsaw puzzles and love to see the picture come together.
- ❍ You love to draw, paint or make things.
- ❍ You're great at building worlds online.

Entertainers

- ❍ You love to sing or play a musical instrument.

- ❍ You love to put on a show.
- ❍ You really feel alive when you dance.
- ❍ You make people laugh and they love to be around you.

Movers

- ❍ You're always on the move.
- ❍ You're happiest doing sport or exercise.
- ❍ You think best when you're doing something: fidgeting, walking or running.
- ❍ You spend lots of time getting better and better at one sport, whether that's football, gymnastics, basketball, baseball or any other.

Imaginers

- ❍ You're a fantastic daydreamer.
- ❍ You love making up games.
- ❍ You could spend hours role playing, where your toys or dolls come to life.
- ❍ You love thinking up new things. Hey presto, you've created a new animal, invented a spaceship or dreamed up a gadget no one's thought of before.

Questioners

- ❍ You love to ask questions, like 'what if?' and 'why not?'
- ❍ Sometimes you challenge how things are done.
- ❍ You love to solve problems others can't.
- ❍ You're brilliant at explaining things. Because you like to find out how things work.

'People' People

- ❍ You're good at understanding how other people are feeling.
- ❍ You can spot how and when to cheer up your friends.
- ❍ You like to help people, it makes you feel happy.
- ❍ You're good at organising things like games and people.

How did you do? Did you find out more about what makes you . . . you? Like many of us, you might be a mix of lots of these things. Or you might shine bright in one main area. The important thing is to discover what makes YOU Xtraordinary and do lots of it, so make the most of your Xtraordinary skills.

There is lots more information in the *Xtraordinary People* book, along with some wonderful illustrations.

Useful links:

Buy our children's book Xtraordinary People, *the perfect resource for explaining dyslexia to children and their teachers, parents, family and friends, here.*

***Watch** our D.Spot vodcast on Dyslexic Superpowers here:*

Do not worry about your difficulties in mathematics. I can assure you mine are still greater.

Albert Einstein

#MadeByDyslexia

DYSLEXIC CHALLENGES

Like dyslexic adults, children Made By Dyslexia find the same things challenging, and this can make school particularly frustrating for dyslexic children. But if spotted early, and given the right support, they can and will do well.

They have trouble learning to read, write and spell as well as remembering lots of facts and figures or concentrating and following instructions. Tests are particularly tricky for dyslexic kids as they are a combination of all these things and can make them feel embarrassed or even stupid, which they are NOT!

So, by far the most important thing we can do for any dyslexic child is to identify their Strengths and place as much importance on them as we do on their Challenges. With help, our kids will learn to do all they need to do well enough, but it's their Dyslexic Strengths that will help them to excel in life.

Early identification and the right support is vital for dyslexic children, so that's why Made By Dyslexia has created our free online dyslexia awareness training films, so parents and teachers around the world can gain the knowledge they need to begin to support their children.

SO, WHAT ARE DYSLEXIC CHALLENGES?

All dyslexics will struggle with some of the following, and the solutions we list will help.

Reading: Difficulties recognising and manipulating sounds, letters and words, make learning to read difficult. Once we've learnt to read, dyslexics will still remain slow readers.

Solution: *Structured, multisensory phonics programmes will enable every dyslexic to learn to read. Extra time in exams, and for assignments, and seeing notes ahead of time make the world of difference. Using devices and assistive technology like speech-to-text and text-to-speech.*

> ***Watch*** *our* 'Dyslexia Awareness: Literacy' *film for lots of amazing tips here:*

Memory systems: Challenges with verbal (remembering verbal instructions), sequential (ordering facts, information), working (keeping facts in mind and manipulating them) and visual (recognising symbols, letters and words) memory make rote learning and getting thoughts down quickly difficult.

Solution: *Support materials include organisers/ planners, mind maps and assistive technology.*

> ***Watch*** *our* 'Dyslexia Awareness: Memory, Organisation and Concentration' *film for lots of amazing tips here:*

Spelling, punctuation and grammar: To be good at spelling, punctuation and grammar you have to learn and retrieve a series of information, skills and rules. Challenges with memory systems make it difficult for dyslexics to learn and apply these rules.

Solution: *Focus on the content of what's being written, not the spelling, punctuation and grammar. Use assistive technology like spellcheck, ask Siri or Alexa, Grammarly and the built-in tools that come with Microsoft and other tech.*

Watch *our* 'Dyslexia Awareness: Dyslexic Challenges' *film for lots of amazing tips here:*

I was an extraordinarily bad speller and have remained so until this day.

Agatha Christie

#MadeByDyslexia

Maths: Challenges with sequential and working memory cause difficulties with learning math facts, times tables and mental maths, although dyslexics are often good at conceptual, high-level maths. So, we often know the answer but cannot tell you how we got there, which is usually required in tests.

Solution: *Look for high-level skills and the skill of 'seeing the big picture' and jumping to the solution. Encourage a love of maths, give support for challenges. Use assistive technology.*

Watch *our* 'Dyslexia Awareness: Maths' *film for lots of amazing tips here:*

Traditional benchmarks: Standardised tests, high-stakes exams in education and many of the psychometric tests used in recruitment disadvantage dyslexics because of all the above.

Solution: *Adjustments and extra time in tests and assignments, project work, exploring different testing methods, use assistive technology, video* *presentations. All will enable dyslexics to demonstrate their real knowledge and skills in order to thrive.*

Watch *our D.Spot vodcast on change-makers to learn more here:*

Watch *our dyslexia awareness film series with tips and strategies from experts on YouTube here:*

Whether you think you can or you think you can't . . . you're probably right.

Henry Ford

#MadeByDyslexia

GROWING UP MADE BY DYSLEXIA – TOP TIPS

We asked parents, kids and teachers from the Made By Dyslexia community around the world to share their top tips, the things they think everyone should know about dyslexia.

Here they are!

PARENTS

1. Your child is brilliant, they just think differently. This thinking is super valuable in the real world.
2. Find their Strengths and passions. Every dyslexic child has Strengths, they may not be super obvious, but they are there.
3. Praise and nurture their strengths at every opportunity and make sure their teachers do this too. This is vital for self-esteem.
4. You know your child better than anyone, so trust your gut when asking for help. Most teachers aren't trained, and many schools don't like to label. Be persistent. Don't give up.

5. Remember their struggles are real, and the sooner they get support, the sooner they can learn, catch up and keep up.

TEACHERS

1. The dyslexia 'label' is a good thing, for teachers, parents and kids. It helps everyone understand their Strengths and Challenges and to give the right intervention.
2. Methods that work for dyslexic kids are actually good for all kids.
3. Never ask a dyslexic child to try harder. They have to work much harder than other kids to learn. Instead, think about how you can change your teaching to make things easier for them.
4. If a child is struggling with spelling, or remembering math facts, or there is a difference in what they can explain verbally and get on paper – think dyslexia.
5. These are brilliant children who don't fit into the traditional education mould. Let them think outside the box and be creative and celebrate their different thinking.

KIDS

1. Don't be worried about being different. Dyslexia gives you lots of Strengths and is a good thing.

2. School can be tough. You will have to work harder than other kids to do the same things. But keep at it, you will get there eventually.

3. Try not to be embarrassed about your dyslexia and the mistakes you make. We're all in the same boat. Struggling with certain schoolwork really isn't the end of the world.

4. All dyslexics have amazing Strengths, things we love to do that are so valuable when we grow up. Find your Superpower and do lots of it. And share it too.

5. Ask for help. Don't suffer in silence. Explain to your teacher, parents and friends what you're finding challenging and ask for help.

Sign up to our Facebook Community to join the conversation.

Key Points

1. There are 7 Archetypes – these are areas that dyslexic children excel in.
2. All children show ability in these, but dyslexic children become 'experts' in them.
3. Focusing on these Strengths builds self-esteem.
4. These Strengths can lead children into careers that are immensely fulfilling and successful.
5. Every dyslexic is different, but we all have Strengths.

The people who are crazy enough to think they can change the world are the ones who do.

Steve Jobs

#MadeByDyslexia

PART 5:

5 Steps to Change

At Made By Dyslexia our mission is to redefine dyslexia. We want to help the world understand and value Dyslexic Thinking, and we have a five-year plan to do that.

If we can redefine dyslexia, and make sure that every school and workplace has trained all staff – then our job will be done. To do that, we need your help. Here are some ways you can join the movement and create change alongside us.

5 WAYS TO MAKE A DIFFERENCE

1. **For EVERYONE – follow us on social media** and join our movement to redefine dyslexia in workplaces, schools and societies, right across the world, by exploring and sharing our content far and wide.

2. **For FAMILIES – watch our videos** and learn how to spot your child's Strengths and nurture them to build self-esteem. Help us kick-start change by asking your school to take our FREE training too.

3. **For KIDS – read *Xtraordinary People*** and watch our films to learn all about Dyslexic Superpowers. Find out what makes you Xtraordinary, and then do lots of it and tell others all about this too.

4. **For TEACHERS – take our FREE training** and learn how to spot, support and empower the one in five dyslexic kids in your classroom. Encourage others to take it too and be a powerful advocate for Dyslexic Thinking in your school.

5. **For EMPLOYERS – get involved with Join the Dots** our workplace initiative with 4 simple steps that will empower Dyslexic Thinking in every workplace and provide an environment where dyslexics thrive. Find out more at www.madebydyslexia.org

5 REASONS WHY WE NEED TO ACT NOW

It's official! Dyslexic Thinking is vital for our future, but that future is closer than we think.

- The fourth industrial revolution is seeing digitisation and AI transforming the skills required in the workplace[1] of the future.
- The skills required for the future (defined by the World Economic Forum) directly map to the Dyslexic Thinking skills.[2]
- The latest research from ManpowerGroup Talent Solutions finds that the pandemic has expedited this change and that in five years, technology will take over 50 per cent of 'human' jobs.[3]
- The remaining 50 per cent of 'human' jobs will require soft skills that are perfectly aligned with Dyslexic Thinking skills.[4]
- We know that 70 per cent of people hide their Dyslexic Thinking from their employer.[5] There are 80 per cent of dyslexic children leaving school with their dyslexia unidentified,[6] yet we have the **exact** skills the future needs. It's time to stand out.

For the good of our children, our businesses and our economies, it's more urgent than ever that we act now.

With your support, we can push governments to ensure that every teacher is trained within five years and guarantee that schools put Dyslexic Thinking at the heart of their curriculums and assessments.

Together, we can lead the charge in workplaces around the globe, as senior leaders, managers, colleagues and employees, redefining dyslexia and helping more people to understand it as a valuable and different way of thinking, which is an asset to EVERY team.

Dyslexia has shaped our past; inventing things we can't live without, helping us make leaps of imagination and discover the unknown. Dyslexia is mission critical to keeping nations safe. It's built brands, created art movements, inspired film-makers, defined world champions and driven change-makers. Its role is vital to our future.

THIS is dyslexia.
And THIS is our time to redefine it, for good.

THIS is dyslexia.
And THIS is our time
to shine. Because the
world needs Dyslexic
Thinking now more
than ever before.
Let your Dyslexic
Thinking stand out
and take your place
in the future.

Kate Griggs

#MadeByDyslexia

References

PART 1: THE BIG PICTURE – INTRODUCTION

1 EY & Made By Dyslexia, 'Value of Dyslexia 1: Dyslexic strengths and the changing world of work', 2018

2 EY & Made By Dyslexia, 'Value of Dyslexia 2: Dyslexic capability and organisations of the future', 2019

3 ManpowerGroup Talent Solutions & Made By Dyslexia 'Seize the D Report', 2021

4 Made By Dyslexia, *Connect The Spots*, 2020

5 BDA, All-Party Parliamentary Group for Dyslexia and other Specific Learning Differences, 'Educational Cost of Dyslexia', October 2019

6 Made By Dyslexia, *Spelling it Out*, 2019

7 BBC Real Story, transmitted on BBC One at 1900 GMT on Wednesday 13 December 2006. See article: http://news.bbc.co.uk/1/hi/programmes/real_story/6175933.stm

8 No To Failure Report, The Dyslexia Sp-LD Trust, 2009

9 Kate Griggs, *Xtraordinary People*, January 2020, published by Penguin Random House Children's

PART 2: THIS IS DYSLEXIA

1 Made By Dyslexia, *Connect The Spots*, 2020

2 Made By Dyslexia, *Spelling it Out*, 2019

3 EY & Made By Dyslexia, 'Value of Dyslexia 2: Dyslexic capability and organisations of the future', 2019

4 Made By Dyslexia, *Connect The Spots*, 2020

5 EY & Made By Dyslexia, 'Value of Dyslexia 1: Dyslexic strengths and the changing world of work', 2018

6 EY & Made By Dyslexia, 'Value of Dyslexia 2: Dyslexic capability and organisations of the future', 2019

7 ManpowerGroup Talent Solutions & Made By Dyslexia 'Seize the D Report', 2021

8 ManpowerGroup Soft Skills Research 2019, ManpowerGroup Talent Solutions Insight 2021. The Future of Jobs Report 2020. World Economic Forum, October 2020

9 Manuel F. Casanova, 'Increased White Matter Gyral Depth in Dyslexia: Implications for

Corticocortical Connectivity.' National Institute of Health, July 9 2016

10 BDA, All-Party Parliamentary Group for Dyslexia and other Specific Learning Differences, 'Educational Cost of Dyslexia', October 2019

11 Made By Dyslexia, *Spelling it Out*, 2019

12 Made By Dyslexia, *Spelling it Out*, 2019

13 Made By Dyslexia, *Spelling it Out*, 2019

14 Made By Dyslexia, *Spelling it Out*, 2019

15 YouGov & Made By Dyslexia, 'Public Perceptions of Dyslexia', April 2017, shared in 'Connecting the Dots, Understanding Dyslexia, Launch Report', May 2017

16 EY & Made By Dyslexia, 'Value of Dyslexia 1: Dyslexic strengths and the changing world of work', 2018

17 EY & Made By Dyslexia, 'Value of Dyslexia 2: Dyslexic capability and organisations of the future', 2019

18 Made By Dyslexia, adapted from 'Value of Dyslexia Report', 2019.

19 Made By Dyslexia, 'Connecting the Dots, Understanding Dyslexia, Launch Report', May 2017

20 Made By Dyslexia, *Spelling it Out*, 2019

PART 3: THIS IS DYSLEXIA IN ACTION

1 Kate Griggs, TEDx Talk, 'The Creative Brilliance of Dyslexia', https://www.youtube.com/watch?v=CYM40HN82I4&t=25s

2 2017 Kauffman Index of Growth Entrepreneurship Ewing Marion Kauffman Foundation

3 Statistic from: https://www.gov.uk/government/news/uks-top-female-entrepreneurs-backed-by-government-to-fire-up-economy-through-innovation

4 Survey commissioned by BBC2 for *Mind of a Millionaire*, source: Ben Flanagan, 'Who wants to be a millionaire?', *The Observer*, October 2003

5 Made By Dyslexia, *Spelling it Out*, 2019

6 Diana Appleyard, 'Education: The art of being dyslexic', *The Independent*, February 1997

7 Made By Dyslexia, *Spelling it Out*, 2019

8 EY & Made By Dyslexia, 'Value of Dyslexia 1: Dyslexic strengths and the changing world of work', 2018

9 EY & Made By Dyslexia, 'Value of Dyslexia 2: Dyslexic capability and organisations of the future', 2019

10 Mari K. Swingle, *i- Minds: How Cell Phones, Computers, Gaming and Social Media Are Changing Our Brains, Our Behaviour and the Evolution of our Species*, New Society Publishers, June 2016

PART 4: THIS IS DYSLEXIA IN KIDS

1 Made By Dyslexia, 'Connecting the Dots, Understanding Dyslexia, Launch Report', May 2017

2 Made By Dyslexia, 'Connecting the Dots, Understanding Dyslexia, Launch Report', May 2017

3 C. Sabey, C. Charlton and S. Charlton, 'The "Magic" Positive-to-Negative Interaction Ratio: Benefits, Applications, Cautions, and Recommendations', *Journal of Emotional and Behavioural Disorders*, March 2018

4 J. Zenger and J. Folkman, 'The Ideal Praise-to-Criticism Ratio', *Harvard Business Review*, March 2013

5 Made By Dyslexia, *Spelling it Out*, 2019

6 Made By Dyslexia, *Spelling it Out*, 2019

7 BDA, All-Party Parliamentary Group for Dyslexia and other Specific Learning Differences, 'Educational Cost of Dyslexia', October 2019

PART 5: 5 STEPS TO CHANGE

1 EY & Made By Dyslexia, 'Value of Dyslexia 2: Dyslexic capability and organisations of the future', 2019

2 EY & Made By Dyslexia, 'Value of Dyslexia 2: Dyslexic capability and organisations of the future', 2019

3 ManpowerGroup Talent Solutions & Made By Dyslexia 'Seize the D Report', 2021

4 EY & Made By Dyslexia, 'Value of Dyslexia 2: Dyslexic capability and organisations of the future', 2019

5 Made By Dyslexia, *Spelling it Out*, 2019

6 BDA, All-Party Parliamentary Group for Dyslexia and other Specific Learning Differences, 'Educational Cost of Dyslexia', October 2019

Kate knows more about dyslexia than anyone I’ve ever met, and to get out there and fight for every dyslexic is just amazing.

Sir Richard Branson

#MadeByDyslexia

About the Author

Kate Griggs is a British social entrepreneur, TEDx Talk speaker and founder and CEO of the transformative charity, Made By Dyslexia.

She is a leading voice in global dyslexia advocacy and has championed a new kind of thinking in the field, which focuses on the strengths of Dyslexic Thinking.

Kate is also the author of children's book, *Xtraordinary People*, the first book to categorise and explain Dyslexic Thinking skills in kids. It became a number one bestseller on Amazon and its groundbreaking new thinking is helping to change the way parents, teachers and children see dyslexia. The charity's celebrity ambassadors, who include Sir Richard Branson and HRH Princess Beatrice, have supported the book in the media.

Made By Dyslexia's purpose is to redefine dyslexia, helping the world to better understand, value and support Dyslexic Thinking. Their mission is to train every teacher in the world by 2030 to spot, support and empower every dyslexic child. And we're empowering every workplace too.

The publication of Kate's new book, *THIS is Dyslexia*, sits alongside the charity's new bold and ambitious global campaign of the same name and is set to redefine dyslexia for good.

Find out more about Kate and the work she does for Made By Dyslexia at www.madebydyslexia.org